The New Dictionary of Symptoms

THE NEW DICTIONARY OF SYMPTOMS

Dr Mike Smith

with Jean Williams

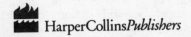 HarperCollins*Publishers*

HarperCollins*Publishers*
77–85 Fulham Palace Road,
Hammersmith, London W6 8JB

A Paperback Original 1993
9 8 7 6 5 4 3 2 1

A catalogue record for this book is
available from the British Library

ISBN 0 586 21312 0

Set in Futura and Meridien

Printed in Great Britain by
HarperCollinsManufacturing Glasgow

CONTENTS

Men's Symptoms

Common Childhood Infectious Illnesses   273

Essential First Aid   279

Medical Diagnostic Tests

FOREWORD

This book is not intended to be a substitute for your own doctor.

Its aim is not to teach you how to diagnose illness but to help you understand more about the common symptoms of ill-health from which we all suffer from time to time.

In recent years, attitudes to health and health care have changed dramatically. Most of us recognize that we play an important part in keeping ourselves well and preventing illness. The importance of a healthy diet and lifestyle is widely accepted.

Being alert to unusual body changes and seeking prompt medical help for certain symptoms can also help avoid ill-health.

Getting appropriate treatment quickly can often stop a small problem from turning into a big nuisance.

Yet most of us are unsure as to when we should seek our doctor's advice and when we can safely ignore minor symptoms and wait for them to clear up on their own. Stomach pain or a cough, for example, can be minor upsets, yet they can also be early warning signs of serious illness. Minor childhood ailments can sometimes cause alarming symptoms, and yet serious illnesses in babies and children can occasionally, in their early stages, appear relatively trivial. When are you safe to wait, and for how long, and when should you get medical help at once?

The New Dictionary of Symptoms helps you to answer these questions.

In it I have set out clearly groups of common symptoms in easy reference sections. I have included sections that deal with the particular health problems of babies, children and pregnant women because I know that these are of special concern to families. Each section will help you identify your symptoms and suggests simple self-help measures where appropriate, or directs you to take medical advice. The type of treatment you might expect to receive if a problem is diagnosed is outlined simply and clearly.

I hope this book will help you in several ways. Firstly, it will direct you to take the right action at home when appropriate and so avoid unnecessary visits to the doctor. It will help you make better use of your time with the doctor if you do need to see him. By being well informed you will be able to ask the right questions and receive fuller answers. Finally, I hope it will reduce some of the fear and anxiety that surrounds illness and ill-health. In my experience ignorance is not bliss when it comes to health matters because much needless worrying is caused by groundless fears.

Note: I've used male terms throughout the book, except in the sections on Women's symptoms and Pregnancy. This is purely for the sake of convenience and is not intended to imply that all patients and doctors are men.

                                                              Dr Mike Smith

INTRODUCTION

In Britain, the majority of people under the age of seventy are fit and well most of the time. Just consider how things have changed for the better even quite recently: forty years ago, the average age of a patient in a medical or surgical ward of a general hospital was around fifty; it's now often over eighty.

For the most part, this improved health into later years has been achieved not by medicines or dramatic new operations (these only come into their own when someone is ill) but rather by the fact that most of us are following an increasingly healthy lifestyle.

The foundation for this is better housing, education and nutrition. Supported by these, we are better placed to understand, choose and then use the healthy options – a balanced diet, regular exercise, and the avoidance of harmful substances like tobacco or excess alcohol.

And since we've become more interested in our own health, both the broadcast and written media now cater for this 'healthy appetite' for information. There have never been more sound facts and opinion readily available about the maintenance of health and the avoidance of disease.

So now, for example, it is possible for most of us to choose to live healthily and disease-free. An individual is especially fortunate if his mother begins by choosing the best time to 'start' him, and opts for a healthy diet and lifestyle even before conception, through pregnancy, and into the early stages of his babyhood. She will now know that it's wise to accept the childhood injections on his behalf, and the offer of a cervical smear, breast examination or blood pressure measurement for herself, as well as the other good things on offer at the ante-natal clinic. In these and other ways we can prevent disease or detect it at such an early stage that it can be controlled or even stopped, once and for all.

Let us not forget that in a developing country, where there aren't the advantages I've mentioned, measles still kills one in ten children – yes, one in ten. Even in Britain, with its 'health foundation', measles can still cause chest and ear problems and an occasional tragedy. But measles will shortly be a disease of the past. All young children are now routinely protected by a vaccine, so the measles virus should soon be eradicated in Britain as the smallpox virus has throughout the world.

And will this progress continue? You bet it will. Apart from those illnesses which can be prevented at source, like smallpox, there will still be others for which our current measures are not enough (for example, stopping smoking will prevent most cancers, but not all). For these and other diseases, the solution lies in our genes.

These 'seeds' are passed on to us by our mothers and fathers at the time of conception. They govern our similarities and differences – how tall we grow, the colour of our skin, eyes and hair – and protect us against some diseases (although they make us vulnerable to others). They can become altered, by chance, at the time of conception or later – it's called mutation – so that, for better or worse, we get a gene that wasn't present in either of our parents. And genes can be altered by pollutants in the environment – certain chemicals, tobacco tars, for example, that can alter the genes to cause a cancer to develop. They can also be altered by a virus – the HIV virus, which alters the genes of certain body cells so that the individual develops AIDS.

Only thirty years ago, most doctors and scientists would never have believed that it would ever be practicable to alter the nature of genes for the better. For a start, they are so small that they can't be seen at all with the strongest light microscope, and in their clumps – chromosomes – only with an electron microscope, which gives tens of thousands times more magnification.

Yet now, using the techniques of genetic engineering, a few genes can be altered. And it seems only a matter of time – and probably not much time at that – before genetic disease will be overcome; and possibly not much more before genes can be manipulated yet more subtly to eradicate even a 'weakness' – a mere susceptibility to a disease such as cancer or heart disease.

So, in writing this book, I am decidedly optimistic that we shall soon be even healthier still. In it, I aim to inform my reader to enable her or him to make better choices about their symptoms, and also about when to call on the pharmacist or other member of a modern health team, such as a health visitor or practice nurse, or to consult their doctor.

The book isn't meant to be a comprehensive aid to diagnosis. That's a doctor's job, and it takes several years of intensive training to acquire the knowledge and skills required. But I hope and believe that you will find this book useful, because most of us are otherwise healthy, and at least nine out of ten of our everyday symptoms will get better, on their own, given time and homely remedies. And this book should help you to recognize the more straightforward symptoms.

The kind of healthy remedies that can help are:

- Extra-warm to hot watery drinks and bed-rest for flu-like symptoms
- Honey and lemon juice, mixed with comfortably hot water, to be sipped for a sore throat or irritating cough
- Weak bicarbonate of soda solution for bathing the surfaces of closed eyelids when the eyes are 'tired' and mildly irritated at the end of a day in a city's polluted air

Beyond that there are a range of 'over-the-counter' medicines that your pharmacist can advise about and supply. Many of these medicines are powerful symptom-relievers. Paracetamol, Ibuprofen or aspirin are all most people will need to relieve everyday pain and inflammatory symptoms. General advice about these is covered in my book *Dr Mike Smith's Handbook of Over-the-Counter Medicines*.

In *The New Dictionary of Symptoms*, I cover everyday symptoms, but also those which are of potentially more sinister importance. So I cannot stress too strongly that if your symptoms are worrying ones, then consult your doctor – even if only for his reassurance. And by worrying symptoms I mean the pain that lasts much longer than you expected, or that changes its nature (for example, what seemed like back-strain has now moved round to the front, and you've developed a temperature).

And worry has to be the criterion that you use – since there is no entirely safe way to give a comprehensive guide to diagnosis to anyone without medical training. And don't knock it. Worry can be a very good guide. Any mother who says of her child 'I'm worried about him; he's not himself' is likely to be on to something, even when a doctor can detect nothing on his first examination.

I suggest that the book will be of greatest service to you as a reference volume, although anyone with an interest in things medical should also find it a good straight-through read. Regular listeners to my broadcasts or readers of my weekly *Woman's Own* column should feel quite familiar with its style. My greatest wish is that it will become a family friend.

GENERAL SYMPTOMS

GENERAL SYMPTOMS

ABDOMINAL PAIN

Abdominal pain can be a sign of disorders associated with the digestive, urinary or reproductive systems. You should always seek your doctor's advice for severe, persistent or recurrent pain.

Severe and continuous abdominal pain needs urgent medical treatment if:

- it goes on for over four hours
- it is unrelieved by vomiting
- it is accompanied by a swollen abdomen
- there is also faintness, drowsiness or confusion

In these cases, if you need to, call an ambulance at once. Don't eat or drink anything while you wait for help in case emergency surgery is needed.

Severe abdominal pain and vomiting or swollen abdomen

When severe pain lasts longer than one hour and vomiting fails to relieve pain, it can be a sign of a serious abdominal condition such as a perforated ulcer or appendicitis. Get medical help at once.

Treatment: You will probably be admitted to hospital for observation and tests, or an exploratory operation may be performed to discover the cause of the pain. If a perforated ulcer or appendicitis is discovered, surgery may be performed to remove the appendix or repair the ulcer.

Pain in the middle of the upper abdomen; comes on after eating

Indigestion is the probable cause of central abdominal pain. This is especially likely following a heavy meal, or if you are anxious or tense.

Treatment: Try to eat meals slowly in a relaxed atmosphere. Eating smaller, more easily digested meals may help. An indigestion remedy from the chemist can relieve the symptoms. If attacks occur often, see your doctor.

Pain in the middle of the upper abdomen, extending up the chest and/or down arms

This may be due to heart pain (see Chest pain, p. 35).

Pain with diarrhoea

Gastroenteritis (inflammation of the digestive tract, see Diarrhoea, p. 51) caused by infection or food poisoning is the most likely cause. You may also have some vomiting.

Treatment: Eat no solid food while the symptoms persist. Drink plenty of clear fluids, water or unsweetened fruit juices. Don't take aspirin or other painkillers. If the symptoms persist for more than two days, consult your doctor.

Severe pain below the ribs on the right

This type of pain can be caused by gallstones. The pain may be very severe and is often accompanied by nausea and vomiting.

Consult your doctor, or, if in severe pain, go to hospital.

Treatment: An injection can be given to relieve severe pain. You will probably be admitted to hospital for tests such as a cholecystography or an ultrasound scan of the gallbladder (see Medical diagnostic tests, pp. 303 and 308).

If gallstones are found, surgery may be necessary to remove them. In some cases, drugs can be used to dissolve the stones.

Pain beginning in the lower back, moving to the groin

A urinary tract infection or kidney stones can cause this type of pain. See your doctor.

Treatment: Your doctor will probably ask for a urine sample for analysis. If an infection is found, you will be prescribed anti-biotics. If kidney stones are suspected, he will arrange for you to have hospital investigations. An intravenous pyelogram (see Medical diagnostic tests, p. 306) may be performed. Kidney stones can be removed surgically or broken up by ultrasound waves using a lithotripter. Advice on diet will be given to help prevent them recurring.

Pain below the waist, urinating more often than usual

An infection of the urinary tract is possible (see Urinary problems, p. 120).

Recurrent abdominal pain

In centre, lower part of the chest
If the pain is relieved by taking antacid medicines, an inflam-mation of the stomach (gastritis) is likely. Alternatively, there may be the possibility of a stomach ulcer.

Treatment: An antacid remedy from the chemist normally helps.

To avoid attacks in future, cut down on smoking and drinking;

both irritate stomach problems. Eat smaller, regular meals and stick to simple foods, not rich or highly spiced. Drink plenty of fluids. If attacks persist despite these self-help measures, see your doctor. He may arrange for a barium X-ray (see Medical diagnostic tests, p. 300) to be undertaken at hospital.

In centre of chest with burning sensation

Hiatus hernia, a condition where part of the stomach protrudes upwards through the chest wall leaking acid juices into the gullet, can cause heartburn and wind. It can be made worse by lying down or bending over, and by being overweight. See your doctor.

Treatment: You doctor will advise taking small, frequent meals and avoiding alcohol and tobacco, which both irritate stomach complaints. He may also advise losing weight if you are too heavy. Antacid and other prescribed medicines can help relieve symptoms. In severe cases an operation to correct the problem can be performed.

With loss of appetite and loss of more than 10 lbs in last two months

A duodenal or stomach ulcer is the most likely cause of these symptoms. However, there is a slight possibility of cancer.

Consult your doctor.

Treatment: Your doctor will probably arrange for tests to be undertaken at hospital. A barium X-ray and/or an endoscopy (see Medical diagnostic tests, pp. 300 and 304) may be performed. If a stomach ulcer is found, you will be given dietary advice and prescribed drugs to control the amount of acid in your stomach. Stomach cancer is usually treated by surgery.

Cramping pain with episodes of diarrhoea and/or constipation

These symptoms may be caused by diverticular disease, where the walls of the large intestine develop 'blow outs' – bulges, like those on the weakened wall of a bicycle tyre – and also become swollen. More commonly they are due to irritable bowel syndrome, which has no obvious cause. This condition is made worse by stress. Anxious people tend to suffer more often than more relaxed types. There is also the slight possibility of bowel cancer. Such symptoms, where they persist, should always be reported to your doctor.

Treatment: Your doctor may arrange tests such as a barium enema (see Medical diagnostic tests, p. 300) to rule out the possibility of bowel cancer. Eating a high-fibre diet is the treatment for both irritable bowel and diverticular disease. An antispasmodic drug may be prescribed to control severe pain. If irritable bowel syndrome is associated with stress or anxiety in your life, learning some relaxation techniques and/or seeking counselling to help resolve problems is worthwhile.

Cramping pain with episodes of diarrhoea

Ulcerative colitis and Crohn's disease both cause these symptoms.

Additionally there may be blood or pus in the diarrhoea. Any such symptoms should be reported to your doctor immediately. Both these conditions are caused by inflammation and ulceration. In Crohn's disease any part of the digestive tract may be affected; in ulcerative colitis only the large intestine is involved.

Treatment: Your doctor will refer you to a specialist for tests.

A barium X-ray and/or a sigmoidoscopy (see Medical diagnostic tests, pp. 300 and 308) will probably be performed. Both disorders may be treated by dietary changes, and anti-inflammatory drugs. In severe cases, surgery may be undertaken to help relieve symptoms, but it cannot always offer a total cure.

Abdominal pain in women

In early pregnancy/with vaginal bleeding
A threatened miscarriage or ectopic pregnancy are possibilities (see Vaginal bleeding in pregnancy, p. 200). See your doctor at once.

**Cramping pains with unpleasant-smelling
vaginal discharge**
An infection of the Fallopian tubes (see Women's symptoms,
p. 186) is a possibility. See your doctor.

Abdominal pain in men

**With swelling or discomfort in the groin, made
worse by coughing or lifting heavy objects**
A hernia is the probable cause of such symptoms. This occurs when
part of the abdomen's contents bulge through a weak area of
muscle in the abdominal wall. See your doctor.

Treatment: If a hernia is confirmed, an operation to repair the
weak muscle-wall may be suggested.

ABNORMAL FAECES

Most changes in the colour or consistency of faeces are due to
changes in diet or a temporary tummy upset. However, certain
changes should be investigated by your doctor since they can be
signs of more serious disorders.

Blood in the faeces

Any blood in the faeces should always be reported to your
doctor.

The most likely cause is haemorrhoids or piles (see Anal problems, p. 25). However, this can also be a symptom of a number
of other disorders such as ulcerative colitis or Crohn's disease
(see Abdominal pain, p. 23). It can also be a symptom of bowel
cancer.

Treatment: Your doctor will probably order tests such as a
barium X-ray or sigmoidoscopy (see Medical diagnostic tests,

pp. 300 and 308) to make a diagnosis. Treatment will depend on what the problem is.

Black or very dark faeces or faeces containing black material

Black faeces are usually caused by eating iron-rich foods such as spinach or beetroot, or by taking iron tablets. They may also be a sign of blood in the faeces caused by bleeding higher up in the digestive tract, possibly from an ulcer. If you have not been taking extra iron in food or tablets, consult your doctor.

Treatment: Your doctor may ask for a sample of faeces and may arrange tests such as an endoscopy or a barium X-ray (see Medical diagnostic tests, pp. 304 and 300). Treatment will depend on the cause of the symptoms.

Very pale faeces

Pale faeces are quite normal for a few days after an infection causing diarrhoea or vomiting. They may occasionally be a symptom of failure to digest or absorb foods, or of a gallbladder or liver problem. See your doctor if abnormally pale – almost white – faeces don't follow a digestive upset.

Treatment: Your doctor will probably take samples of blood and faeces for analysis. Further tests may be needed to make a diagnosis. Treatment will depend on the cause of the problem.

ANAL PROBLEMS

Bleeding from the anus

Haemorrhoids, or piles, is the most likely cause of such bleeding. These are swollen veins around the anus. They may be aggravated by constipation and often occur during pregnancy and after child-birth. See your doctor.

Treatment: Your doctor will examine you. If he diagnoses haem-orrhoids, there are several types of treatment. You may be pre-scribed cream or suppositories to shrink the haemorrhoids. If they are particularly troublesome, they can be treated by a hospital specialist with injections to shrink them, or by freezing or 'band-ing'. This technique involves placing a tight band around the swollen vein which then gradually withers away.

Occasionally surgery will be advised.

Avoiding constipation by eating a high-fibre diet and drinking plenty of fluids can help enormously. Constipation aggravates the condition by putting extra pressure on the veins. If it is avoided, haemorrhoids may disappear without any further treatment.

Wart-like lumps around the anus

Anal warts can be caused by a viral infection. See your doctor.

Treatment: Your doctor will probably refer you to a skin clinic.

Warts may be removed by freezing, by applying a lotion, or surgically under local anaesthetic.

Itching around the anus

When this itching has no obvious cause, it is described as pruritus ani.

Treatment: Self-help measures such as washing with plain water twice a day, avoiding scented soaps and bath products that may irritate, and resisting the urge to scratch, may help.

Additionally, wear cotton underpants only next to the skin and avoid tight clothing. A soothing ointment can help.

Itching around the anus, white threads in faeces

Threadworms cause such symptoms. These are harmless parasites which are easily passed from person to person. Children are often affected.

Treatment: If you have children, check them for signs of thread-worms. Do they complain of an itchy bottom, especially first thing in the morning, or at night? Look at their faeces before flushing the loo. And, if they aren't embarrassed by it, gently separate the cheeks of their buttocks and check their anus for the presence of worms. Treat the whole family (even those who have no obvious signs of infection) at once with a proprietary medicine from the chemist. Follow the instructions exactly. You will probably need to repeat the dose again in a couple of weeks.

Meanwhile, ensure that all the family scrupulously wash their hands in hot water with soap after every visit to the lavatory.

ANXIETY

Anxiety may be a temporary response to a stressful situation or it may be a long-term difficulty. It can express itself in both emotional and physical ways. The anxious person may feel tense, stressed, fearful and have a constant sense that something awful is about to happen. He may worry about his own health or that of family and friends. He may also suffer physical symptoms such as panic attacks with breathlessness, chest pains, palpitations, headache, backache, stomach pains, insomnia, lack of appetite and tiredness.

There are many theories about the nature of anxiety. Some doctors believe that a difficult childhood and/or an unsatisfactory or unhappy relationship with parents predisposes a person towards anxiety. Others believe that anxiety is a reaction to too much stress or difficult life events such as job loss, divorce or bereavement. There are two main approaches to its treatment. Anti-anxiety drugs and anti-depressants, on some occasions, can help minimize distressing symptoms and allow the person to cope better. They do not, however, tackle the source of long-standing or recurrent problems. Therapy, counselling or psychoanalysis are more long-term solutions which attempt to help the anxious person overcome anxiety by understanding the reasons for it and by providing some skills to help him cope.

Anxiety following a major upset such as divorce, bereavement, redundancy

The stress caused by such an upset can cause considerable anxiety.

Treatment: Self-help measures such as minimizing stress in other areas, not taking on new responsibilities or commitments, taking life quietly, and paying attention to eating well and getting enough rest, can help. Try to avoid drinking or smoking more than usual, as doing so will put the body under more strain. Make an effort to spend time in relaxing activities you enjoy – sport, reading, gardening, for example – rather than just slumping in front of the television. If the anxiety is severe enough to stop you coping with everyday life, consult your doctor.

Anxiety caused by giving up smoking, drinking, sleeping-pills or tranquillizers

Withdrawal symptoms from these drugs may include anxiety and other physical symptoms such as trembling and insomnia.

Treatment: Seek your doctor's advice for help with withdrawal symptoms. It's possible he may prescribe a short course of drugs to help overcome anxiety while reducing dependency. He will also be able to put you in touch with one of the self-help organizations that offer support to those wishing to give up cigarettes, drink or other drugs. These groups provide invaluable advice and practical help; they can be of great assistance.

Anxiety in social situations

This is a very common problem which often eases as the sufferer gains more experience of meeting and mixing with others.

If such anxiety prevents you from enjoying a full social life, consult your doctor.

Treatment: A mild anti-anxiety drug may be prescribed to help overcome the problem in the short term. The doctor may suggest therapy or counselling if the problem is severe.

Anxiety about specific situations or objects

A phobia or compulsive disorder, of which there are many types, may be the cause of anxiety. Some people have a fear of enclosed spaces (claustrophobia) or a fear of being outdoors (agoraphobia), for example, or they have an irrational fear of things or places such as supermarkets or churches, cats or spiders, which prevents them from leading a normal life.

Treatment: Your doctor may prescribe an anti-depressant or anti-anxiety drug to help you cope with your phobia. He may recommend counselling or psychotherapy to help you overcome the anxiety.

Anxiety about sex

This is common at all stages in life. Many people, from teenagers to those in much later life, worry about sex for different reasons. If the fear or worry cannot be resolved by a frank and sympathetic discussion with your partner, seek your doctor's advice.

Treatment: Your doctor will discuss the problem with you and may be able to offer help and advice. If he feels you need more help he may refer you for sex counselling.

BACK PAIN

Most people suffer from backache from time to time. It is often brought about by unaccustomed exercise or by awkward bending, lifting or stretching. Such movements can fatigue the muscles, strain or damage the ligaments that hold the vertebrae and discs between them together, or even damage the intervertebral discs.

In later life, general wear and tear on the spine and degenerative diseases due to ageing may be the cause of back pain. Severe pain can result from pressure on the spinal nerve when the vertebrae are misaligned or damaged.

Severe pain after strenuous exercise or heavy lifting

If the pain is bad enough to stop you moving, or if it shoots down one leg, a prolapsed (slipped) disc is possible. This happens when awkward or unaccustomed movement or strain causes one of the jelly-like discs between the vertebrae to bulge.

Treatment: Resting flat on your back in bed and taking painkillers while the pain persists is the best treatment. If the pain becomes more severe or is no better after twenty-four hours, call your doctor. He may arrange for you to have tests, or he may simply prescribe more rest, stronger painkillers and possibly manipulation of the spine.

In severe cases of prolapse, surgery may be recommended.

Severe pain following an injury or fall

If the pain is accompanied by difficulty moving your arms or legs, or by tingling or loss of bladder or bowel control, you should call an ambulance. Damage to the spinal cord is possible. Keep still and warm while you are waiting.

Treatment: Examination and X-rays will be carried out to discover what damage has been done. Treatment will depend on the result of these investigations. Rest may be sufficient to allow healing, but in some cases surgery may be required.

Moderate pain or aching after strenuous exercise or lifting

You may have strained or bruised some of the muscles or ligaments in the back, especially if the activity is unaccustomed.

Treatment: Follow the advice outlined above and call your doctor if there is no improvement in twenty-four hours or if the pain becomes severe.

Stiff lower back and/or hips developing over months or years in middle age

An inflammatory disease of the joints between the vertebrae (ankylosing spondylitis), which can develop in later life, is possible. It causes the spine gradually to become stiff and inflexible and may also be painful. A second condition, lumbar spondylosis (the name given to changes that take place in the lower back as a result of wear and tear), is also a possibility. A loss of disc material and cartilage between the vertebrae can make the spine stiff and painful.

Consult your doctor.

Treatment: Your doctor will probably arrange X-rays of your back and pelvis and also blood tests if he suspects ankylosing spondylitis. This condition is sometimes treated with injections of anti-inflammatory drugs to reduce pain and stiffness. The main treatment for both conditions is regular gentle exercise such as swimming or yoga to help strengthen the muscles of the back. You may be referred to a physiotherapist for specialist help.

Stiff back in middle age with pain mainly between shoulder blades

Arthritis of the bones in the neck (cervical osteoarthritis) due to wear and tear as you get older is a possible cause of this pain. It may also cause pain in the arms and shoulders, numbness and tingling in the hands, and a weak grip. Consult your doctor if symptoms become worse or troublesome.

Treatment: X-rays or other tests may be undertaken. Severe neck pain may be treated with rest, painkillers, heat treatment, supporting the neck in a collar, or physiotherapy.

Sudden severe pain in later life

A sudden compression of a vertebra (crush fracture) as a result of osteoporosis (thinning of the bones) is possible, especially in women who suffer far more often from osteoporosis than men.
Consult your doctor.

Treatment: Your doctor will arrange for you to have X-rays if he suspects a fracture. In the meantime, he will prescribe pain-killers. A crush fracture will heal of its own accord in time. For women, if osteoporosis is diagnosed, your doctor may offer hormone replacement therapy (HRT), which slows down bone loss, and advise you to eat a calcium-rich diet. Men will be offered dietary advice.

Pain in lower back on one side, feeling generally unwell

A kidney infection, especially if you have a high temperature, is likely. Consult your doctor at once.

Treatment: Your doctor will ask for a specimen of urine. If he suspects a kidney infection, he will probably prescribe antibiotics right away.

BREATHING DIFFICULTIES

Sudden severe difficulty with breathing, especially when accompanied by a bluish tinge around the mouth, is a medical emergency. Get help at once. Any serious breathing difficulty should be reported to your doctor since there is a possibility that it may threaten the body's oxygen supply. Breathing difficulty accompanied by pain in the chest suggests a problem affecting the heart (see Chest pain, p. 35). See also Wheezing, p. 130, for other problems relating to breathing.

Breathlessness with temperature of 38° C (100° F) or above and/or cough

A chest infection such as pneumonia or bronchitis can cause such symptoms. These are both dangerous illnesses, especially in the elderly or those in poor health. See your doctor at once.

Treatment: Your doctor will prescribe antibiotics. He may advise hospital admission in severe cases.

Sudden attack of breathlessness, especially at night, coughing white or pink frothy phlegm

A build-up of fluid in the lungs is possible. This can be dangerous. Call your doctor at once or go to hospital. Sit up to make breathing easier while you wait for help.

Treatment: You will probably be admitted to hospital and be given oxygen and drugs to help your breathing. Long-term treatment will depend on the cause of the problem.

Sudden attack of breathlessness, coughing blood, especially after being in bed due to illness, surgery or pregnancy

A blood clot in the lung (pulmonary embolism) is a possibility.
This is a life-threatening condition. Get medical help at once.

Treatment: You will probably be admitted to hospital. Specialist tests such as chest X-ray, radioisotope scan of the lungs and electrocardiography (see Medical diagnostic tests, p. 299) will be carried out. If a blood clot is found, you will be given drugs to dissolve it and to prevent any more forming.

Breathlessness and cough with thick greenish-yellow phlegm

Chronic bronchitis (inflammation of the airways of the lungs) is possible, especially if you smoke and have suffered previous bouts of coughing with phlegm. See your doctor.

Treatment: You will probably be sent for a chest X-ray. Your doctor will prescribe antibiotics and possibly an inhaler to help widen the air passages. If you are a smoker, he will urge you to give up and perhaps suggest that you get some help to enable you to do this.

Breathlessness at times of stress

Severe anxiety can cause attacks of breathlessness (see Anxiety, p. 27).

Breathing difficulty while eating

It's likely that the sufferer is choking on a piece of food. This can be a medical emergency. Carry out the first-aid procedures described on p. 290 if the person isn't able to cough up the obstruction in his windpipe.

CHEST PAIN

Most chest pain is due to minor problems such as indigestion or pulled muscles. However, severe, crushing chest pain, or pain associated with breathlessness or irregular heartbeat, can be a sign of a serious disorder of the heart or lungs and may need emergency treatment.

Sudden gripping or crushing pain spreading from the centre of the chest to the arms or neck

If the pain persists in spite of several minutes' rest, a heart attack is a possible cause. Get medical help at once.

Treatment: Loosen tight clothing and stay calm while waiting for help. Admission to hospital, where monitoring and resuscitation equipment is available if needed, is likely. Strong painkillers and oxygen will probably be given in the first instance. Other drugs to prevent blood clots and to control disturbances of the heart's rhythms may also be administered.

Heart attacks are caused by the build-up of fatty deposits in the arteries which reduce the flow of blood to the heart. Long-term treatment includes changes in diet and lifestyle and probably taking one or more drugs to reduce the likelihood of further attacks.

Mild to severe chest pain, sensation of pressure in centre of chest, sweating, dizziness, breathlessness

These symptoms are typical of angina, due to not enough oxygen being carried to the heart muscle. Angina tends to occur during times of stress or exertion and, unlike a heart attack, the pain is generally relieved by rest. It is usually caused by a build-up of fatty deposits in the arteries which gradually reduce the flow of blood to the heart.

See your doctor immediately.

Treatment: Your doctor may arrange for you to have tests such as electrocardiography (ECG) (see Medical diagnostic tests, p. 304). If angina is confirmed, you will be given drugs to help prevent and relieve attacks.

Sudden attack of chest pain and breathlessness and/or coughing blood, especially after being in bed due to illness, surgery or childbirth

A blood clot in the lungs (pulmonary embolism) is a possibility.

Get medical help at once.

Treatment: You will probably be admitted to hospital where you may be given tests such as a chest X-ray, radioisotope scan of the lungs and/or electrocardiography (ECG) (see Medical diagnostic tests, p. 299) to confirm the diagnosis. If a blood clot is found you will be given drugs to help dissolve it and to prevent any more forming.

Chest pain and cough with thick greenish-yellow phlegm

Acute bronchitis (inflammation of the airways of the lungs) is possible.

Treatment: Take painkillers if there is discomfort, drink plenty of fluids, and stay in a warm environment. If there is no improvement after forty-eight hours, or if you become breathless, see your doctor.

Chest pain and breathlessness with temperature of 38° C (100.4° F) or above and/or cough

A chest infection such as pneumonia or bronchitis can cause such symptoms. These are both dangerous illnesses, especially in the elderly or those in poor health. See your doctor at once.

Treatment: Your doctor will prescribe antibiotics. He may advise hospital admission in severe cases.

Pain in centre of the lower chest with burning sensation

Hiatus hernia, a condition where part of the stomach protrudes upwards through the chest wall leaking acid juices into the gullet, can cause heartburn and wind. It can be made worse by lying flat or bending over and by being overweight. See your doctor.

Treatment: Your doctor will advise taking small, frequent meals and avoiding alcohol and tobacco which both irritate stomach complaints. He may also advise losing weight if you are too heavy. Antacid and other prescribed medicines can help relieve symptoms. In severe cases an operation to correct the problem can be performed.

Pain in the middle of the chest, comes on after eating

Indigestion is the probable cause of this type of pain. It is especially likely following a heavy meal, or if you are anxious or tense.

Treatment: Try to eat meals slowly in a relaxed atmosphere.

Eating smaller, more easily digested meals may help. An indigestion remedy from the chemist can relieve the symptoms. If attacks happen often, see your doctor.

Chest pain with coughing and/or shortness of breath/fever/sweating at night

Tuberculosis (TB), a lung infection, can cause these symptoms. TB is comparatively rare in developed countries, but is more common in deprived city areas, among the elderly and those suffering from diabetes or disorders of the immune system. See your doctor.

Treatment: If your doctor suspects TB he will ask for a sample of phlegm for analysis. He will send you for a chest X-ray at hospital. If the diagnosis is confirmed, treatment is a long course of antibiotics. Most patients make a full recovery within a few months with no lasting effects.

Burning pain in skin, not affected by breathing

Shingles, a viral infection of the nerves, is a possibility. The pain will be followed in about five days by a blistery rash. If possible, see your doctor before the rash appears.

Treatment: An antiviral drug to limit the illness can be given in the early stages, provided diagnosis is made quickly.

Painkillers and soothing skin ointment will probably be given.

The blisters normally dry out and heal after two to three weeks, but unfortunately pain may persist for some weeks or months in about a third of cases.

CONFUSION AND FORGETFULNESS

Everyone suffers from confusion and forgetfulness occasionally, especially if preoccupied or under stress. This is usually no cause for concern. However, sudden or severe symptoms should always be brought to the attention of your doctor.

Confusion and/or forgetfulness following head injury

A blow or injury to the head can cause bruising of the brain.

Mild confusion shortly after the injury is usually no cause for concern, but severe confusion that develops some days later may indicate bleeding within the skull. See your doctor if you suffer any kind of head injury.

Treatment: If your doctor suspects brain injury he will refer you to hospital for a full examination and X-ray of the skull. If bleeding inside the skull or a fracture is found, surgery may be needed.

Confusion or forgetfulness and/or numbness and tingling in any part of the body/blurred vision/difficulty speaking/loss of movement in arms and legs

A stroke due to disruption or a temporary interruption of the blood supply to the brain can cause these symptoms. Strokes are rare in people under sixty, but the chances of having one increase rapidly with age after this. If symptoms last for less than a day and disappear completely, the episode is known as transient ischaemic attack. See your doctor at once.

Treatment: You may be treated at home or sent to hospital, depending on the severity of the attack. In cases of mild stroke, you may be given drugs to control high blood pressure if this is a problem, and referred to a physiotherapist for help if movement has been lost.

In more severe cases, hospital investigations such as a CAT scan, ECG (electrocardiography), chest X-ray or angiography (see Medical diagnostic tests, p. 299) may be undertaken to discover the extent of any damage to the brain and to rule out other problems. Drugs may be prescribed to prevent recurrence and therapy offered to help restore any loss of movement or speech.

Confusion in diabetics

An attack of hypoglycaemia (too little glucose in the blood) is likely. This occurs when the delicate balance between insulin and food intake is upset, for example if a meal is delayed, or unaccustomed exercise taken.

Treatment: Give the sufferer a hot sweet drink immediately, or, if this is not available, any quickly absorbed source of sugar – some sweets, a fizzy drink, or a bar of chocolate. If recovery does not start within ten minutes, call medical help immediately.

Confusion and forgetfulness developing gradually over a period of months and/or personality changes/inability to cope with everyday things/decline in standards of appearance and hygiene

Senile dementia, a common disorder in later years causing the brain to stop functioning normally, is possible. Seek medical help.

Treatment: If senile dementia is diagnosed, your doctor will offer advice on how to cope with the problem and refer you to sources of help and support available in the health service.

Confusion and forgetfulness due to drugs or alcohol

Excessive consumption of alcohol can cause confusion and memory loss as well as other unpleasant symptoms. Certain pre-scribed drugs, particularly anti-anxiety drugs, can also cause these problems. See your doctor if drugs or alcohol cause behaviour changes you are unhappy about.

Treatment: Depends on the cause of the problem.

CONSTIPATION

There is no rule that proclaims that everyone should open their bowels once a day. For some people twice or more times a day is normal; for others, once every two days or more is enough. Constipation is suffered only when faeces are hard and painful to pass, or less frequent than normal. A great many cases of constipation respond to an increase in fluids and fibre in the diet. Very few of us eat as much fibre as dietary guidelines recommend (30 gms (1 oz) per day) or drink enough water (at least 4 pints).

Fibre intake can be increased by eating more high-fibre foods such as:

• wholemeal bread and cereals
• fruit and vegetables
• beans, peas, lentils and other pulses

A second very common cause of constipation is putting off the urge to defecate because it's not convenient at the time. If the urge to open the bowels is constantly resisted it can lead to a loss of normal bowel reflexes. Making a conscious effort to use the lavatory whenever the 'call' is felt can help to restore reflexes to normal.

Over-use of laxatives can, paradoxically, cause constipation by making the bowel inactive. Stopping their use and eating extra fruit and high-fibre foods should be enough to restore normal function. You should never routinely dose yourself with laxatives.

Constipation with cramping pain in the lower abdomen

Irritable bowel or diverticular disease (see Abdominal pain, p. 22) can cause such symptoms. See your doctor if several episodes of pain and constipation occur within a few months.

Treatment: If your doctor suspects a bowel illness he will arrange for you to have tests such as a barium enema or a sigmoidoscopy (see Medical diagnostic tests, pp. 300 and 308). Treatment involves adopting a high-fibre diet. Drugs may also be prescribed.

Constipation after taking medicines

Opiate-based painkillers like codeine, cough mixtures containing codeine, any medicines containing morphine or iron and other drugs such as antacids, some anti-depressants and tranquillizers can cause constipation. Increase your fibre and fluid intake to help overcome the problem. If you are persistently constipated, seek your doctor's advice.

Treatment: Your doctor may advise further dietary changes, or he may change your medication or prescribe a laxative to help overcome the problem.

Painful defecation

Haemorrhoids (piles) or a small tear in the lining of the anus (anal fissure) can cause painful defecation (see Anal problems, p. 25).

COUGHING

Coughing is the body's natural response to an irritant, such as the mucus produced by a cold, in the throat or lungs, or to fumes or smoke in the atmosphere. Occasionally it can be a symptom of a more severe disorder.

Dry cough producing no phlegm

A dry cough with no phlegm and no other symptoms that lasts for over a month should be reported to your doctor. It is probably due to an allergy or to smoking, but there is a slight possibility that it could be due to a more serious disorder such as a growth in the windpipe, or to lung cancer.

Treatment: Your doctor will consider your symptoms and may arrange for tests to determine if there is any underlying problem causing the cough. He may ask for samples of blood for analysis.

A chest X-ray or a bronchoscopy (see Medical diagnostic tests, p. 302) are two further tests he might arrange to be undertaken in hospital. Treatment will depend on the cause of the problem.

Cough with thick yellow or green mucus and/or wheezing/high temperature, following a cold

Acute bronchitis, often a complication of a cold or flu, is likely. Usually this clears up naturally within three or four days. If it persists longer, or in the case of an elderly person, a baby, a heavy smoker or a person with lung disease, call the doctor.

Treatment: Keeping warm indoors, drinking plenty of fluids and inhaling steam can help reduce symptoms. A doctor will check for any complications, and may possibly prescribe antibiotics.

Persistent cough with thick greenish-yellow mucus produced every day, wheezing, breathlessness

Chronic bronchitis is possible, especially if you tend to suffer from this type of cough every winter. This disease is an inflammation of the airways and lungs most often due to smoking.

See your doctor.

Treatment: Your doctor may order tests such as a chest X-ray or an analysis of the mucus to see how badly you are affected. He may prescribe antibiotics to help clear lung infection or an inhaler to help breathlessness by moistening the air and widening the airways. He will strongly advise you to give up smoking which is, these days, the main cause of the illness.

Cough with runny nose and/or sore throat

A common cold, an infection of the nasal passages, is the most likely cause (see Runny nose, p. 91).

Cough with high temperature and breathlessness

Pneumonia, a potentially dangerous infection of the lungs, is a possibility. Call your doctor at once.

Treatment: Your doctor may prescribe antibiotics. Severe cases may require hospital admission.

Chest pain with coughing and/or shortness of breath/fever/sweating at night

Tuberculosis (TB), a lung infection, can cause these symptoms. TB is comparatively rare in developed countries but is more common in deprived city areas, among the elderly and those suffering from diabetes or disorders of the immune system. See your doctor.

Treatment: If your doctor suspects TB he will ask for a sample of phlegm for analysis. He will send you to have a chest X-ray in hospital. If the diagnosis is confirmed, treatment involves a long course of antibiotics. Most patients make a full recovery within a few months with no lasting effects.

DEAFNESS

Complete deafness is very rare and is usually present from birth.

Partial deafness, which may come on suddenly, or over a period of time, is usually the result of infection or blockage of the ear due to wax, injury to the ear, or worsening hearing due to age.

Gradual hearing loss over several weeks

A build-up of wax in the ear is the likely cause of such hearing loss.

Treatment: On no account try to remove ear wax by poking anything into your ears. Eardrops from the chemist can be used to soften the wax which may then run out, or fall out as a plug. If the wax doesn't come away like this, see your doctor, who will syringe it out.

Gradual hearing loss in older people

The natural degeneration of hearing with age affects some people more than others. It can cause sounds to become less clear and create a problem understanding speech. See your doctor.

Treatment: Your doctor will arrange for you to have a hearing test. A hearing aid helps most people overcome this problem.

Sudden hearing loss with sticky yellow discharge from ear and/or earache

An ear infection is probably the cause of deafness. See your doctor.

Treatment: Your doctor will probably prescribe antibiotics as tablets, eardrops, or an injection to clear up the infection.

Hearing will return to normal once the infection has cleared.

Loss of hearing with runny nose, sore throat, catarrh

The eustachian tube linking the throat and ears is probably blocked because of a cold. This should resolve itself as the cold gets better and needs no specific treatment. Consult your doctor if hearing isn't back to normal within a week.

Gradual loss of hearing due to exposure to loud noise

If you often listen to very loud music at rock concerts, disco-theques or through headphones, or if your work involves fre-quent exposure to loud noise, your hearing could be permanently damaged. Make every effort to prevent further damage by wear-ing earplugs or ear defenders if you do noisy work. Avoid listen-ing to loud music through headphones or standing close to speakers at concerts. See your doctor if hearing loss is a problem.

Treatment: Your doctor will arrange for you to have hearing tests. A hearing aid can help.

Hearing loss with sudden attacks of dizziness and/or nausea/ ringing in the ears

Ménière's disease is a possibility if you are over fifty. This disorder is caused by too much fluid in the inner ear canal that controls balance. It usually only affects one ear. Attacks of dizziness may last only minutes or continue for many hours. See your doctor.

Treatment: Your doctor will probably arrange hearing tests to diagnose the disorder. He will advise you to rest in bed during an attack and may suggest that you cut down your salt intake. A drug to reduce the nausea and other symptoms may be pre-scribed.

DEPRESSION

Depression is a word that's often used to describe a general sense of feeling low and down in the dumps. We all suffer from such feelings from time to time, and they are usually an entirely normal response to the stresses and disappointments of everyday life. However, such feelings coupled with other symptoms such as anxiety, mood swings, loss of appetite, trouble sleeping, loss of interest in sex and social life, constant tiredness and lack of energy, are signs of a depressive illness that needs treatment.

Some 10 to 15 per cent of people suffer depression at some time in their life. More women than men are affected, and depression becomes more common with increasing age.

Depression can be brought about by distressing events or illness, and there are certain times of life when depression is more likely — after having a baby, for instance (see Depression after childbirth, p. 195), during adolescence or middle age. Often in true depressive illness there is no single obvious cause. Depression can be a symptom of a wide range of psychiatric illnesses.

Depression for no apparent reason, sleeping poorly, no appetite, feelings of hopelessness, despair, guilt, worthlessness

These are symptoms of severe depressive illness. Consult your doctor at once.

Treatment: There are three main types of treatment for depression: psychotherapy, drugs and ECT (electroconvulsive therapy). Depending on the severity of your illness, a doctor may prescribe drugs, or refer you to a counsellor or to a hospital specialist for treatment.

Psychotherapy, either individually or in a group, is thought to be especially useful for patients whose personality or life experiences are the main cause of their problem. This might include an unhappy or difficult childhood, problems relating to others, difficulty forming or maintaining relationships, or disturbing events or changes in life. Drug treatment is often used for patients whose symptoms are mainly physical. Anti-depressant drugs, unlike tranquillizers, are not addictive. ECT (electroconvulsive therapy), given only in hospital under general anaesthetic, is reserved for treating severely depressed people, or those who have failed to respond to other types of treatment.

Depression following bereavement

Depression can be a very normal part of the grief that accompanies a bereavement. A period of mourning is a very necessary part of coming to terms with the loss of a loved one.

It may take as much as two years before the bereaved feel able to participate in life again. Denying or blocking distressed or unhappy feelings is not helpful. It prevents the bereaved person progressing through their grief. If you are afraid that feelings of grief and sadness will overwhelm you, or if depression is preventing you from coping with everyday life, your doctor may be able to prescribe anti-depressant drugs to give some temporary help. More long-term help may be found by contacting an organization such as CRUSE – Bereavement Care (see Useful addresses, p. 330), which has trained counsellors and a nationwide support system.

Depression following viral illness such as flu or glandular fever

Infectious illnesses are often followed by a period of feeling low. Rest as much as you need to and try to eat well and get lots of sleep to recover your strength. If the depression lasts longer than a month, or you are finding it very distressing, consult your doctor.

Depression due to strain at work or home

General stress due to feeling under pressure can cause depression. Try to find a close friend, relative or colleague who you can confide in and who will help you to make some decisions about how best to deal with your problems. Be sure to eat well, get enough rest, and try to avoid too much drinking or smoking.

Try to spend some time each day relaxing, exercising, or doing something you enjoy to take your mind off pressing worries for a short while. If these measures do not help, or the depression seems to get worse, consult your doctor.

Depression due to divorce, job loss or other distressing event

Depression due to distressing events in life is called 'reactive depression'. Some people cope better than others with such problems. If depression is preventing you from coping with everyday life, consult your doctor.

Treatment: Your doctor may prescribe anti-depressants to help get you over a bad patch. If depression lasts longer than a few weeks, or you are severely depressed, he may refer you for specialist help.

Depression during the winter months

Seasonal affective disorder (SAD) is a rare form of depression which is thought to be due to not getting enough hours of daylight. It's true also that the colder weather and lack of sun curtail people's activities and social life and this in itself may lead to low spirits. Some SAD sufferers find relief by using 'daylight' bulbs or fluorescent tubes (which mimic natural light) for a few hours each day during the winter months. Most people who suffer from SAD find that it disappears spontaneously in the spring when the days become longer.

Depression following drinking

Many people do not realize that alcohol has a depressant effect on the body. This effect may last even on those days when no drink is taken. If the depression persists despite cutting down or cutting out alcohol, or if you find it difficult to do without drink, consult your doctor.

Depression in middle age or later years

Depression becomes more common with increasing age. This is due to circumstances such as children leaving home, career difficulties or disappointments, health problems or fear of old age. In women the menopause can often lead to periods of depression (see Absent periods, p. 171). Self-help measures such as confiding in close friends or relatives, taking up a new hobby or activity, making an effort to re-evaluate one's role in life and to accept the ageing process, can all help. If you cannot cope with the depression see your doctor for help.

Depression in women before a period

Many women become miserable, irritable or depressed before a period, feelings which usually disappear as soon as bleeding starts. If you find pre-menstrual depression hard to cope with, or if it is affecting your life, consult your doctor.

Treatment: No single method of treatment has proved completely effective, but measures such as drugs to relieve fluid retention, progesterone supplements, dietary changes (for example, avoiding salt, caffeine and chocolate and taking vitamin B6 or evening primrose oil) have proved effective with some women.

Depression after childbirth

Depression after the birth of a child is very common (see Depression after childbirth, p. 195).

DIARRHOEA

Diarrhoea is not itself an illness but rather a symptom of an underlying problem, and is usually no cause for concern except in the elderly, those who are already ill, and babies who can become dangerously dehydrated very quickly (see Babies under one, p. 207).

The most common cause of diarrhoea is food poisoning due to eating food contaminated with bacteria or viruses. However, frequent attacks of diarrhoea can be a symptom of a more serious problem of the digestive tract and should be investigated by a doctor.

Diarrhoea with nausea and/or vomiting/high temperature

Gastroenteritis (inflammation of the digestive tract) due to food poisoning is the most likely cause.

Treatment: Most mild attacks of food poisoning last only two or three days. Resting in bed, taking frequent, small amounts of clear fluids (water or unsweetened fruit juices, not milk), and only gradually beginning to take bland foods when the symptoms have subsided, is usually all that's needed. Pharmacy-supplied mineral replacement drinks can bring quicker relief.

The sufferer should pay special attention to hygiene while he's ill, wash hands thoroughly with hot water and soap after using the lavatory, avoid sharing towels or face-flannels, and discontinue preparing food, to prevent infecting other family members. Taking anti-diarrhoea medicines is not routinely recommended since they can prolong the illness. If there is no improvement within two days see your doctor.

Cramping pain with episodes of diarrhoea and/or constipation

These symptoms may be caused by diverticular disease, where the inner lining of the large intestine bulges outwards (diverticulates) through its walls – like a blowout or bulge on the weakened wall of a bicycle tyre. More commonly, they are due to irritable bowel syndrome which has no obvious cause.

This condition is made worse by stress. Anxious people tend to suffer more often than more relaxed types. There is also the slight possibility of bowel cancer. Any change in bowel habit lasting more than two weeks should always be reported to your doctor.

Treatment: Your doctor may arrange tests such as a barium enema (see Medical diagnostic tests, p. 300) to rule out the possibility of bowel cancer. Eating a high-fibre diet is the treatment for both irritable bowel and diverticular disease. An antispasmodic drug may be prescribed to control severe pain. If irritable bowel syndrome is associated with stress or anxiety in your life, learning some relaxation techniques and/or seeking counselling to help resolve problems is worthwhile.

Several episodes of diarrhoea with blood or mucus in the faeces and/or cramping abdominal pains

Ulcerative colitis and Crohn's disease both cause these symptoms. Blood in the faeces should always be reported to your doctor immediately. Both these conditions are caused by inflammation and ulceration of the digestive tract. In Crohn's disease any part of the digestive tract may be affected; in ulcerative colitis only the large intestine is involved.

Treatment: Your doctor will refer you to a specialist for tests. A barium X-ray and/or a sigmoidoscopy (see Medical diagnostic tests, pp. 300 and 308) will probably be undertaken. The main treatment for both disorders is dietary change and anti-inflammatory drugs. In severe cases surgery may be performed to help relieve symptoms, but it cannot always offer a cure.

Repeated attacks of bloody diarrhoea with abdominal pain/vomiting and high temperature

If you have recently travelled abroad you may have contracted dysentery. This is a serious infection of the digestive tract. See your doctor at once.

Treatment: There are two types of dysentery. Diagnosis is made by taking a sample of faeces for testing. The main risk with both types is dehydration and the spread of infection. Mild cases may be treated at home. More serious infections may need hospital treatment. Antibiotics and other drugs may be administered.

EARACHE

Earache is generally caused by an infection which is usually quite simply treated. Earache is far less common in adults than in children.

Earache with a cold and a blocked-up nose

A cold that produces a lot of mucus and blocks the nasal passages can sometimes cause mild earache.

Treatment: Painkillers can help relieve symptoms. A wrapped hot-water bottle held against the ear may be comforting. If the pain persists for more than three days, or becomes severe, see your doctor. He may prescribe a decongestant or antibiotics if there is infection.

Earache with blocked-up feeling in ear and/or sticky discharge

An ear infection, perhaps as a result of the eustachian tube linking the ear and throat becoming blocked, is possible. See your doctor.

Treatment: Your doctor may prescribe decongestant drops or spray to clear the blockage, and/or antibiotics.

Earache and blocked-up feeling during or after an aircraft flight

The air pressure balance between the middle and outer ear can be disturbed by flying. Pinching the nostrils and blowing the nose can be enough to restore normality. If the problem persists for more than a day or two, consult your doctor.

Earache with blocked-up feeling in ear/loss of hearing

A build-up of wax in the ear is the likely cause of earache and hearing loss.

Treatment: On no account try to remove ear wax by poking anything into your ears. Eardrops from the chemist can be used to soften the wax. Then try lying in a warm bath with your ears submerged to loosen it. It the wax doesn't come away like this, see your doctor, who will syringe it out.

FAINTNESS AND FAINTING

Faintness, a sensation of light-headedness together with feeling cold and clammy or pale, sometimes followed by momentary loss of consciousness, is caused by a sudden drop in blood pressure which reduces the blood supply to the brain. This may be due to a shock, or to low blood sugar.

Fainting and feeling faint often occur during early pregnancy (see Pregnancy and childbirth, p. 196). It can happen after getting up suddenly from sitting or lying down and is sometimes caused by going for too long between meals and getting very hungry. Prolonged exposure to hot sun can also cause fainting.

Faintness can be dealt with by lying down with legs raised up high, or by sitting with the head between the knees to restore blood flow to the brain. Open windows if the room is stuffy and loosen tight clothing. If a person loses consciousness for more than a few minutes, or if breathing slows, becomes noisy or irregular, call medical help at once.

Usually, feeling faint or fainting is nothing to worry about, but if you are often affected, or have other symptoms too, you should see your doctor.

Faintness with numbness and tingling and/or blurred vision/trouble speaking/confusion/loss of movement in arms or legs

A stroke due to disruption or a temporary interruption of the blood supply to the brain can cause these symptoms. Strokes are rare in people under sixty, but the chances of having one increase rapidly with age after this. If symptoms last for less than a day and then disappear completely, the episode is known as a transient ischaemic attack. See your doctor at once.

Treatment: You may be treated at home or sent to hospital, depending on the severity of the attack. In cases of mild stroke, you may be given drugs to control high blood pressure if this is a problem, and referred to a physiotherapist for help if movement has been lost.

In more severe cases, hospital investigations such as a CAT scan, ECG (electrocardiography), chest X-ray or angiography (see Medical diagnostic tests, p. 299) may be undertaken to determine the extent of any damage to the brain and rule out other problems. Drugs may be prescribed to prevent recurrence and therapy offered to help restore any loss of movement or speech.

Faintness in diabetics or because of hunger

An attack of hypoglycaemia (too little glucose in the blood) is likely. This happens when the delicate balance between insulin and food intake is upset, for example if a meal is delayed, or unaccustomed exercise taken. In other cases it's usually because of going too long between meals. Headaches, dizziness, feelings of weakness, and trembling are also possible.

Treatment: Give the sufferer a hot sweet drink immediately, or if this is not available any quickly absorbed source of sugar — some sweets, a fizzy drink or a bar of chocolate. If recovery does not start within ten minutes in diabetics, call medical help immediately.

Faintness with slowing down or speeding up of heartbeat

Any sudden disturbance of the heart rate can cause dizziness or faintness due to a reduction in the blood supply to the brain.

Slowing or speeding up of the heartbeat can be a perfectly normal response to stress. At times, however, it may also be a sign of an underlying heart problem. See your doctor.

Treatment: If your doctor suspects a heart problem he may refer you to hospital for tests such as ECG (see Medical diagnostic tests, p. 304) to check your heart rate and electrical activity. Abnormal heart rhythms may be treated with drugs or in some cases by fitting a pacemaker to maintain normal heartbeat.

FEVER

A fever is usually regarded as a temperature of over 38° C (100° F). It is generally the body's response to bacterial or viral infections. A raised temperature helps to protect the body by killing off the invading cells. Fever may be accompanied by symptoms such as sweating, shivering, headache, and fast breathing. If fever lasts longer than two days, or if your temperature rises above 40° C (104° F), you should consult your doctor.

High temperature with runny nose and/or sore throat/headache/aching limbs

A viral infection such as flu is likely.

Treatment: Stay in bed, drink plenty of fluids, and take aspirin or paracetamol to reduce fever and help aches and pains. If you become breathless, or if there is no improvement within two days, call your doctor.

High temperature with shortness of breath even when resting and/or coughing up yellow or green mucus

These are symptoms of pneumonia, which can be a serious illness, especially in the elderly or those not in good health. Call your doctor.

Treatment: Mild cases of pneumonia can be treated at home. Your doctor will probably suggest that you take aspirin or paracetamol to reduce fever and inflammation, and prescribe antibiotics. More serious cases may require hospital treatment.

High temperature with wheezing and coughing up yellow or green mucus

Acute bronchitis may be a possibility, especially if you've had a cold or flu.

Treatment: Drink plenty of fluids and take aspirin or paracetamol to reduce fever. If there is no improvement within two days, call your doctor.

High temperature with severe headache and/or stiff neck/nausea or vomiting/drowsiness or confusion/dislike of bright lights

Meningitis, an inflammation of the membranes surrounding the brain, can cause such symptoms. This is a dangerous illness. Call your doctor at once.

Treatment: You will probably be admitted to hospital. Diagnosis will be confirmed by taking a sample of fluid from the spinal cord by lumbar puncture (see Medical diagnostic tests, p. 306). Treatment for bacterial meningitis is antibiotics often given by drip. For viral meningitis, the less severe form of the illness, no specific form of treatment is necessary other than painkillers and extra fluids.

High temperature with pain in the lower back and/or pain when passing urine/frequent need to urinate/pink or cloudy urine

An infection of the bladder or kidney can cause these symptoms. Call your doctor.

Treatment: Your doctor will ask for a urine specimen and will probably prescribe antibiotics. If he suspects an underlying kidney problem, he may arrange special tests such as intravenous pyelography (see Medical diagnostic tests, p. 306).

High temperature with lower abdominal pain and/or heavy or unpleasant-smelling vaginal discharge

An infection of the Fallopian tubes (salpingitis) is possible (see Women's symptoms, p. 186).

Consult your doctor.

Treatment: Your doctor will probably take a sample of vaginal discharge for analysis and prescribe antibiotics.

FOOT PROBLEMS

Painful, aching or irritated feet are not usually a sign of any serious problems. They are most likely to be caused by not taking good care of your feet or by wearing ill-fitting shoes.

Itching between the toes; soft, red, peeling skin

Athlete's foot, which is a fungal infection, can cause such symptoms. Sometimes the fungus also affects the nails and makes them thick and yellow-looking.

Treatment: Effective anti-fungal creams, powders and sprays for athlete's foot can be bought at the chemist's. The virus thrives in warm, moist conditions, so keep your feet as dry as possible.

Always dry feet thoroughly between toes after washing. Wear cotton socks to absorb moisture and avoid plastic shoes or boots that make the foot sweat. If the condition doesn't clear up within a few weeks, see your doctor. He may prescribe stronger anti-fungal cream or tablets.

Hard lumps of skin on toes or sides of feet

Corns and calluses are caused by pressure from new or badly fitting shoes and can become very painful.

Treatment: If badly fitting shoes are causing the problem, changing to a better-fitting pair will stop it. In the meantime, corn solvents bought at the chemist's can soften hard skin. Corn plasters, little spongy rings, can ease pressure on painful areas. If corns give persistent trouble, treatment from a chiropodist, who will also give advice on foot care, will help.

Painful lump at the base of big toe

A bunion is an inflamed fluid-filled pad that covers the side of a deformed joint at the base of the big toe. It can become inflamed and very painful. Bunions are usually caused by a lifetime of wearing badly fitting shoes.

Treatment: Make sure that all your shoes fit properly and don't put additional pressure on the bunion. If it becomes very painful or inflamed, consult your doctor. In extreme cases an operation to straighten the big toe is performed.

Pain and tenderness in corner of nail on big toe

An ingrown toenail is possible. Cutting the big toenails down in the corners, or wearing badly fitting shoes, can cause ingrown toenails which may then become infected and painful.

Treatment: Always cut your toenails straight across. Don't leave splinters of nail or jagged edges at corners. Wear shoes that fit well and don't press the toes together. If an ingrown toenail becomes painful, see your doctor.

Pain in sole of foot with patch of thickened red skin and/or black speckles

A verruca is likely. This is a type of wart which is caused by a virus (see Moles and warts, p. 71).

Pain in sole of foot with inflamed, red area

An infection, perhaps from a cut or wound, or a piece of glass stuck in the foot, is possible. See your doctor.

Treatment: Your doctor will remove any foreign body he finds in the foot. He may prescribe antibiotics if there is any infection.

GIDDINESS

Feeling giddy for no obvious reason may be a symptom of several types of disorder.

Giddiness with confusion and/or numbness and tingling in any part of the body/blurred vision/difficulty speaking/loss of movement in arms and legs

A stroke due to disruption or a temporary interruption of the blood supply to the brain can cause these symptoms. Strokes are rare in people under sixty, but the chances of having one increase rapidly with age after this. If symptoms last for less than a day and disappear completely, the episode is known as a transient ischaemic attack. See your doctor at once.

Treatment: You may be treated at home or sent to hospital depending on the severity of the attack. In cases of mild stroke you may be given drugs to control high blood pressure if this is a problem, and referred to a physiotherapist for help if movement has been lost.

In more severe cases hospital investigations such as a CT scan, ECG (electrocardiography), chest X-ray or angiography (see Medical diagnostic tests, p. 299) may be undertaken to determine the extent of any damage to the brain and rule out other problems. Drugs may be prescribed to prevent recurrence and therapy offered to help restore any loss of movement or speech.

Giddiness with loss of balance and/or vomiting

An inflammation of the inner ear due to viral infection (labyrinthitis) may cause these symptoms. See your doctor.

Treatment: Your doctor will examine your ears and if labyrinthitis is diagnosed may prescribe drugs to help calm the symptoms. You will be advised to rest quietly in bed until the condition clears up.

Attacks of giddiness with hearing loss and/or nausea/ringing in the ears

Ménière's disease is a possibility if you are over fifty. This disorder is caused by too much fluid in the inner ear canal that controls balance. It usually only affects one ear. Attacks of dizziness may last only minutes or continue for many hours. See your doctor.

Treatment: Your doctor will probably arrange hearing tests to diagnose the disorder. He will advise you to rest in bed during an attack and may suggest that you cut down your salt intake. A drug to reduce the nausea and other symptoms may be prescribed.

Attacks of giddiness with feelings of acute anxiety and/or breathlessness/racing heart/dry mouth

A panic attack due to being in a situation which causes you acute anxiety is possible (see Anxiety, p. 27).

HAIR AND SCALP DISORDERS

The condition of your hair is dependent upon overall good health.

Periods of ill-health or stress or a poor diet may cause dull, thin or brittle hair. Harsh hairdressing methods such as perming, bleaching, drying or curling with fierce heat can damage your hair. Additionally, there are a number of specific disorders which affect the growth and condition of the hair.

Thinning hair/hair loss

Some hair loss is almost inevitable as we grow older. In men, the pattern of hair loss is largely inherited. In women, the loss of female hormones after the menopause can cause some thinning of the hair. Noticeable hair loss is very common between three and six months after childbirth and sometimes happens after stopping the contraceptive pill. It can also be the result of a long or serious period of ill-health or chemotherapy treatment for cancer.

Treatment: Any sudden hair loss for unexplained reasons should be reported to your doctor. Hair loss due to childbirth or stopping the contraceptive pill is only temporary. The hair should return to normal within a few months. Normally, hair lost because of chemotherapy will begin to re-grow once treatment finishes.

However, if there is extensive or distressing hair loss during treatment, help with a wig or a hair-piece is normally available.

Thinning, dry hair with tiredness/weight gain/ feeling cold often

These can be symptoms of hypothyroidism, a condition in which the thyroid gland fails to produce enough hormone. This problem is most common in middle-aged women. See your doctor.

Treatment: Your doctor may take tests to diagnose the condition, or he may send you to a hospital specialist. Treatment for under-active thyroid is with tablets of thyroxine to replace the natural hormone the body is failing to produce. The tablets need to be taken for life in the same way that diabetics need to take insulin every day. Most patients feel much better soon after treatment begins, and return to normal within a few months.

Bald patches developing suddenly

A fungal infection such as ringworm can cause patchy hair loss.

It may also cause the scalp to be sore and itchy. A condition known as alopecia areata may also suddenly create bald patches. The cause of this is not well understood. It is thought in some cases to be related to emotional stress.

Treatment: Anti-fungal shampoo, creams or tablets can be pre-scribed by the doctor to treat ringworm. There is no specific treat-ment for alopecia areata. Generally, the first attack clears up and new hair begins to grow within six to nine months.

Intensely itchy scalp

Head lice or nits can cause severe itching. Check your scalp behind the ears and at the nape of the neck. Any tiny brown insects or white gritty flakes like dandruff indicate head lice are present.

Treatment: Ask your chemist to recommend a suitable shampoo or lotion. Treat the whole family at the same time, since head lice are very contagious. Head lice are commonly caught by children at school. Their presence does not indicate any lack of hygiene; on the contrary, head lice like clean hair. Combing the hair regularly with a fine-toothed nit comb to dislodge any eggs before hatching is the best protection against re-infestation.

HEADACHE

Most people suffer a headache from time to time. It is usually caused by tension, tiredness, hunger, drinking too much alcohol or being in a hot, smoky or stuffy room for too long. The vast majority of headaches are not a symptom of any serious disorder and clear up within a few hours. However, a severe headache that lasts for longer than a day, especially with other symptoms such as nausea or vomiting, or frequent headaches that happen several times a week, should be reported to the doctor.

Headache with high temperature

Many infectious illnesses, like colds and flu, cause fever and headache (see Fever, p. 57).

Headache with blocked nose

This is often a symptom of colds. However, colds can sometimes cause inflammation of the mucus membranes lining the sinuses, the air-filled cavities in the bones around the nose. Sinusitis can cause a throbbing ache or pain around the nose and eyes and usually thick catarrh that blocks the nose and affects the sense of smell. Some people suffer bouts of sinusitis after every cold.
   Treatment: Staying in a warm, humid atmosphere helps.
   Inhalations of warm steam (add a drop of menthol and eucalyptus inhalation to the water if preferred) three or more times

a day relieve symptoms and can help clear the sinuses. Take paracetamol or aspirin (not under twelve years) for the discomfort. If you are no better within two days, see your doctor. He may prescribe decongestants or antibiotics. A minor operation to clear the sinuses is sometimes recommended for people who suffer persistently with sinusitis.

Severe headache with nausea or vomiting/ severe throbbing pain on one or both sides of forehead and/or blurring or loss of vision

An inflammation of the arteries in the head, temporal arteritis, is a possibility, especially if you are over fifty. This is quite a rare disorder and affects more women than men. Call your doctor at once.

Treatment: Your doctor may wish to take a blood test to confirm the diagnosis. He will probably prescribe steroid drugs to reduce inflammation. These may need to be taken long-term, and you will be monitored at regular intervals if this is the case.

Severe one-sided headache with nausea or vomiting and/or blurred vision

Migraine affects about 10 per cent of the population and is three times more common in women than men. Migraine headaches may be triggered by certain foods such as cheese, chocolate and red wine, or they may be brought about by tension, or by loud noise and bright or flickering lights. Many women find that menstruation or the contraceptive pill trigger migraine headaches.

Treatment: Take paracetamol or aspirin to relieve pain and rest quietly in a darkened room until the attack has passed. Try to discover what triggered the headache and avoid it in future. If migraines happen more than once a month, see your doctor. He may prescribe drugs to help prevent further migraines.

Dull aching headache in and above the eye/ blurred vision and/or nausea or vomiting

Acute glaucoma, a serious disorder in which pressure builds up in the eye, is a possibility, especially if you are over forty. Call your doctor at once.

Treatment: Your doctor will prescribe eyedrops and possibly other drugs to reduce the high pressure in the eyeball. Usually surgery is necessary a little later to prevent the problem happening again.

Headache after reading or doing close work like sewing

Strain on the neck muscles as a result of poor posture or great concentration while working can cause a tension headache.

Treatment: Take paracetamol or aspirin to relieve the pain. A hot drink or a soak in a warm bath may help to relieve tension. Good light, directed from behind and onto the activity, and a comfortable, well-supported chair, may help prevent tension headaches in future.

Headache following blow or injury to the head

A blow to the head that causes bruising, or a more serious injury that causes bleeding in the brain or damage to the skull, is possible if the headache doesn't clear up within a few hours. If you vomited or felt sick, were confused, unconscious or lost your memory, even for a short while after the incident, seek medical help at once, by attending a hospital casualty department or calling an ambulance if necessary.

Treatment: You will be fully examined and X-rayed. Treatment depends on the nature of the injury but may include surgery.

HOARSENESS

Hoarseness or loss of voice is nearly always caused by an inflammation of the voice box (larynx). Laryngitis may be short-lived and over in a few days, or it may be chronic and persist for far longer.

A viral illness such as a cough, cold or sore throat can often cause loss of voice, a dry, irritating cough and painful throat.

Using the voice a great deal, especially over a long period, can cause the vocal cords to become persistently inflamed. Smoking and heavy drinking can also lead to chronic laryngitis. Follow these self-help measures to treat loss of voice:

- Rest the voice as much as possible, and that includes whispering – don't
- Take paracetamol or soluble aspirin for the discomfort
- Take plenty of warm drinks to keep the throat moist
- Avoid smoking and alcohol

If there is no improvement within four days, or if you start to cough phlegm, see your doctor. He will probably prescribe a course of antibiotics for the infection.

Persistent loss of voice that lasts for longer than two weeks or keeps recurring should always be checked by your doctor.

Occasionally this can be a sign of cancer of the larynx.

LUMPS AND SWELLINGS

Lumps or swollen areas suddenly appearing beneath the skin are usually the result of the lymph glands responding to infection.

The lymph glands are situated all over the body, but those near the surface, in the neck, under the arm, and in the groin, are most often noticed if they become swollen. They will usually be rather tender and slightly warm lumps.

Occasionally, swollen lumps under the skin are caused by a sebaceous gland becoming blocked or by an abscess.

Any painful, persistent or worrying swelling should always be referred to your doctor. For lumps or swellings in the breasts, see Breast problems, p. 156.

Lumps or swellings in the neck, armpit or groin with high temperature/sore throat/tiredness/ headache/feeling generally unwell

Glandular fever, a viral infection that affects the lymph nodes – often called glands – is possible. This illness is particularly common among teenagers. Consult your doctor.

Treatment: If glandular fever is suspected, your doctor will probably take a blood test to confirm the diagnosis. Treatment of glandular fever involves rest, plenty of fluids and paracetamol or soluble aspirin to reduce discomfort. It may take several months to make a full recovery. Tiredness and lack of energy often persist even once the main symptoms have subsided.

If the blood test fails to confirm glandular fever, other sources of infection may be looked for. There are many other conditions which can cause enlarged lymph nodes in the body.

Several chronic infections, such as brucellosis – a rare disease usually caught from infected milk – or a virus transmitted by a scratch from a cat – an even rarer condition called cat-scratch disease – will all be considered as a diagnosis. Also, leukaemia, a cancer of the blood, will be an uncommon cause which the doctor will need to consider together with equally serious conditions such as AIDS.

Lumps or swellings under jaw and/or high temperature/headache/ painful throat

Mumps, an infectious viral illness usually caught by children, is a possibility (see Common childhood infectious illnesses, p. 277).

Painful, tender red swelling anywhere on the body

A boil caused by a bacterial infection is possible. This can arise anywhere on the body except the palms of the hands and the soles of the feet. When it is larger, an abscess caused by a bacterial infection is possible. An abscess forms when pus collects beneath the surface. The gums and breasts are common sites for abscesses, but they may occur anywhere on the body. See your doctor.

Treatment: Antibiotics may be prescribed to fight the infection.

Your doctor may possibly lance the boil or abscess to release the pus and ease pain.

Soft lump in the groin that disappears when pressed

Hernias cause such lumps, especially in men. They occur when a weakness in part of the abdominal wall allows part of the abdomen's contents to protrude. See your doctor.

Treatment: If the hernia is causing discomfort, your doctor may recommend surgery to repair the abdominal wall.

Lumps or swellings near an infected cut or wound

The lymph glands near the site of a wound may sometimes swell as they respond to the infection.

Treatment: Clean the wound with cotton wool and clean water or a mild antiseptic solution. Cover with a sterile dressing. If the wound is pussy, painfully inflamed, or if the gland is still swollen after the wound has healed, consult your doctor.

Smooth, painless pale lump beneath the skin

A cyst in a sebaceous gland is likely, especially if the lump is on the scalp, face or ears. The gland can become filled with thick 'cheesy' fluid. Although harmless unless they become infected and sore, sebaceous cysts can look unsightly.

Treatment: See your doctor if a cyst becomes red or sore. If the lump is ugly, it may be removed under local anaesthetic either in a hospital outpatients clinic, or at your doctor's surgery.

MOLES AND WARTS

Warts are the result of a viral infection. Moles are caused by too much pigment being produced in the skin and an overgrowth of certain skin layers. Warts and moles are generally entirely harmless. However, in some instances troublesome moles can be an early warning of skin cancer which is very easily treated at this stage. For this reason, any changes in appearance should be referred to your doctor. See your doctor if a mole:

- bleeds
- changes colour
- becomes larger
- itches

Your doctor will refer you to a specialist if he has any doubts.

The specialist, if cancer is considered possible, will take a sample of tissue for biopsy, and the mole will be removed, by freezing or surgery under local anaesthetic, depending on its size and site. When necessary, a skin graft will be used to replace the skin removed.

Small, hard raised lumps, pink or white with rough surface

Common warts are caused by a virus which makes skin cells grow rapidly. They are caught by touch or by contact with skin cells shed from a wart. They can appear anywhere on the body. On the feet they are known as plantar warts or verrucas.

Treatment: Warts usually disappear naturally within a month or so, and it is best to leave them alone to do this if possible.

However, if warts are causing trouble or are unsightly, see your doctor for treatment.

Verrucas also tend to disappear naturally over time. However, if they are painful, see your doctor or a chiropodist for treatment. Children who are prone to picking up verrucas from swimming-pools and showers can get protection by wearing rubber 'verruca socks' which prevent contact with the virus in the damp environment where it thrives.

Warts around the anus or genitals

Genital warts are caused by exactly the same virus as those elsewhere on the body. They can be more irritating, though, because the skin is more sensitive in this area. For this reason, don't attempt to treat warts in this area yourself. See your doctor.

Treatment: Your doctor will prescribe a cream or paint to use on the wart. He will usually advise avoiding sexual contact until the warts have cleared, since they can be spread in this way.

NAIL PROBLEMS

There are several problems which may affect the growth of the nail. Although these may be unsightly or irritating, they are not usually harmful or dangerous.

Discoloured, thickened or flaky finger or toenails

This problem is usually caused by a fungal infection. Thick and flaky nails, especially on the toes, tend to affect older people more often, although it is not really clear why.

Treatment: Although this problem is not easy to clear up, your doctor may prescribe a course of anti-fungal tablets or cream which can help in some cases.

Brittle, flaky fingernails

A tendency to brittle nails is made worse by exposure to water, detergents or harsh chemicals.

Treatment: Wear protective gloves whenever nails are in water – apart from personal 'toilet' – or exposed to chemicals. Applying hand cream will often help.

Pitted and thickened nails

The skin disorder psoriasis, which causes patches of flaking, scaly skin all over the body, can also affect the nails like this.

In bad cases the nails can also become loosened or lifted from the nail-beds. See your doctor.

Treatment: There are many treatments for psoriasis, including various drug treatments, soothing creams and exposure to ultra-violet light.

NUMBNESS AND TINGLING

Numbness and tingling, usually known as 'pins and needles', is caused by a temporary disturbance of the nerve impulses to the brain. It usually happens after an arm or leg has been held in an awkward position for a while. Persistent numbness or tingling that occurs for no apparent reason should be investigated by your doctor.

Numbness and tingling in hands/weak grip/ pain in the arms and shoulders/stiff neck

Cervical spondylitis, a disorder of the joints between the vertebrae in the neck, can put pressure on the nerves of the arms and hands and cause tingling and numbness. This disorder is most common in people over fifty. See your doctor.

Treatment: Your doctor may arrange an X-ray to check on the diagnosis. Heat treatment, rest, a surgical collar to support the neck, physiotherapy and painkilling drugs are all used in the treatment of this disorder.

Numbness and tingling in fingers/shooting pains in wrists, worse at night

Carpal tunnel syndrome, a disorder in which swelling of the tissues in the wrist puts pressure on the main nerve there, can cause these symptoms. The problem is especially common in pregnant as well as middle-aged women.

Treatment: The disorder sometimes rights itself without treatment – especially after pregnancy. However, if it is persistent or troublesome, see your doctor. He may refer you to a specialist to confirm the diagnosis. Anti-inflammatory drugs, or wearing splints at night, can help the condition and, in persistent cases, surgery can be performed to relieve pressure on the nerve.

Numbness and tingling on one side of the body only and/or weakness in arms or legs/blurred vision/confusion/trouble speaking/loss of movement in arms or legs

A stroke or a transient ischaemic attack may both cause these symptoms. Both involve a disruption of the blood supply to the brain. If you have any of the symptoms listed above, or think you may have suffered a stroke, call your doctor at once.

Treatment: Treatment depends on the severity of the attack. In some cases none may be necessary, or the doctor may refer you to hospital for specialist tests such as a CAT scan or electrocardiogram (see Medical diagnostic tests, pp. 303 and 304). Treatment depends on the results of such tests.

Numbness and tingling in fingers and toes in cold weather/pain when feeling returns

Raynaud's syndrome is a disorder which causes the small blood vessels that serve the fingers and toes to contract suddenly in cold weather and cut off the blood supply. The fingers go white and then become red and painful as the blood supply is restored.

Treatment: Keep the hands and feet as warm as possible in cold weather. Avoid smoking; this constricts the blood vessels even further. If the problem is very painful, consult your doctor. In some cases, drugs to relax the walls of the blood vessels may be prescribed.

OVERWEIGHT

It's estimated that between 30 and 35 per cent of the UK population is overweight. About 5 per cent, those who weigh more than two stones over their maximum desirable weight (see Ideal weight charts, p. 313), are obese. Being overweight progressively increases a person's chances of becoming seriously ill with high blood pressure, stroke, coronary heart disease, diabetes or arthritis. Disorders such as cancer of the colon and rectum in men and cancer of the breast, uterus and cervix in women are associated with overweight.

Becoming overweight is nearly always the result of eating too much food for the body's energy needs. In a very small number of cases, a hormonal imbalance, hypothyroidism (see Tiredness, p. 115), can cause weight increase. However, it's irritating but true that a tendency towards obesity is mainly inherited. The children of obese parents are ten times more likely to become obese than children with parents of normal weight. It seems that some of us can eat too much and get away with it, at least for a while, but others can't.

Obesity is on the increase in our society and it's likely that many of us have a low energy requirement because of our inactive lifestyles. We put on extra weight because we simply eat too much for our needs. However, there are certain circumstances that increase the risk of gaining excess weight:

- Growing older. After the age of forty, the body begins to take longer to burn up food. This may also be accompanied by taking less exercise as we age
- Giving up smoking. This is often accompanied by a temporary weight gain of up to 5 lbs, usually due to extra eating to compensate for lack of cigarettes
- During pregnancy. A woman's body uses food more efficiently though there is often a tendency to 'eat for two'
- When depressed. Some people compensate for feeling low by eating extra food for comfort
- Changing from a physically active to a more sedentary job or lifestyle

How to lose weight

Most experts are agreed that, to lose weight, changes to diet must be gradual and permanent. 'Crash' diets that give dramatic weight loss in weeks very rarely provide a permanent solution to overweight because about 60 per cent of dieters put back all the weight they lose eventually. It is much better to make small steps towards reducing your calorie intake, substituting low-fat spread for butter, semi-skimmed milk for full-cream, sweeteners for sugar, for example – changes that you can stick to. Changing the balance of the type of foods you eat, cutting down on high-calorie fats and sugars and boosting your intake of fresh fruits and vegetables, can form the basis of a weight-reducing diet.

Here are some dietary guidelines:

Cut out or severely reduce your intake of: butter, cream, full-fat cheeses, ice cream, alcohol, sugar, sausages, pies, cakes, pastries, chocolate, bacon, fried foods, sweetened cereals, thick sauces and gravies, puddings, jam, honey, syrups, sweet and fizzy drinks

Reduce your intake of: beef, lamb, pork, eggs, whole milk, pasta and rice, thick soups, bread

Eat as much as you like of: non-oily fish, poultry, salads, fresh fruit and vegetables, unsweetened fruit juice

Making these changes should result in noticeable weight loss within one month. Consult your doctor for help if you fail to lose weight with these changes in eating habits.

PAIN IN FACE

Facial pain is usually caused by infection or inflammation.

Although it can be very uncomfortable it is rarely a sign of a serious disease.

Facial pain with or following a blistery rash

Shingles, a viral infection of the nerves to the skin, could be a possibility, especially if you are over fifty. See your doctor at once; prompt treatment can limit the severity of the illness.

Treatment: If shingles is in its early stages, the doctor may prescribe an antiviral drug. Otherwise an ointment and/or painkillers may be offered. The blisters associated with the illness should clear within three weeks. Unfortunately, pain from damage to the nerve endings may persist for weeks or, in a few cases, months or even years.

Pain in cheek bones or around eyes with or following cold, worse when bending forward

Sinusitis, an inflammation of the air cavities in the skull (sinuses), can cause such symptoms.

Treatment: Stay inside in a warm, humid atmosphere. Take soluble aspirin or paracetamol to relieve discomfort. Inhaling steam from a basin several times a day can help. Decongestant nosedrops may also give some relief, but are not to be used for more than five days except on a doctor's instructions. If there is no improvement within four days, see your doctor. He may prescribe antibiotics.

Severe pain behind one eye

Cluster headaches, a type of migraine, can cause this symptom (see Headache, p. 65).

Brief, severe stabbing pain on one side of face only

Trigeminal neuralgia, a disorder of the trigeminal nerve of the face, can cause severe pain in the cheeks, gums, lips or chin on one side of the face. The pain is over very quickly but is severe while it lasts. This problem is unusual in people under fifty.

A similar type of pain can also be caused by infections of the ears, teeth or sinuses.

Treatment: See your doctor. A prescribed medicine can bring considerable relief. Painkillers can also help, and in severe cases, a minor operation might be considered.

Severe throbbing pain on one or both sides of the head, especially the temples

Temporal arteritis, an inflammation of the arteries within the scalp, can cause this type of pain. This is a rare illness which usually affects older people only (see Headache, p. 66). Consult your doctor without delay, since urgent treatment with steroid medicines is essential to protect the eyesight.

PAINFUL ARM

Pain in the arm is usually due to straining or spraining muscles or ligaments after unusual or strenuous activity – playing a sport for the first time in ages, for example. If you rest the arm, pain will usually disappear within a few days. See your doctor if the pain is persistent or recurs.

Severe pain after an injury or fall, even when resting/unable to move arm

A fracture or serious injury to muscles or ligaments is possible.

Call an ambulance or get to hospital as quickly as you can. Avoid moving the injured arm; this may do further damage. Strap or tie it securely across your chest. Don't eat or drink anything before you set off to hospital in case surgery is necessary.

Treatment: An examination and probably an X-ray will be undertaken. An operation to set the bone may be necessary. Depending on the damage, the arm may need to be plastered, splinted or held in a firm bandage while it heals.

Pain after strenuous exercise, an injury, violent movement or fall

A strain or sprain of the muscles or ligaments in the arm and/or bruising is probably causing the pain.

Treatment: Apply an ice-pack to the injury. This will reduce inflammation and swelling. Bandage the arm firmly but not too tightly. Take aspirin or paracetamol to reduce pain. Rest the arm as much as possible during the next week. If the pain is severe, or no better within twenty-four hours, see your doctor.

Pain in the shoulder or upper arm when moved

An inflammation of the shoulder joint caused by injury or sprain is likely.

Treatment: Rest the arm as much as possible. Take aspirin or paracetamol to reduce pain. See your doctor if there is no improvement within three days.

Pain down the arm/numbness in hand, especially first thing in the morning

Pressure on the nerve as a result of the carpal tunnel syndrome, a constriction caused by a tough band of fibres at the wrist – the carpal tunnel.

Treatment: Wearing wrist splints in bed at night may bring temporary relief. However, an orthopaedic surgeon may need to operate to relieve the constriction.

Pain down the arm or in the shoulder/numbness and tingling in hands/weak grip/stiff neck

Cervical spondylitis, a disorder of the joints between the vertebrae in the neck, can put pressure on the nerves of the arms and hands and cause pain or tingling and numbness. This disorder is most common in people over fifty. See your doctor.

Treatment: Your doctor may arrange an X-ray to check on the diagnosis. Heat treatment, rest, a surgical collar to support the neck, physiotherapy and painkilling drugs are all used in the treatment of this disorder.

Pain down the arm and/or chest pain

There is a possibility that this pain could be caused by angina (see Chest pain, p. 35).

Pain down arm and pins and needles in hand, worse at night and first thing in the morning

These symptoms can be caused by carpal tunnel syndrome (see Numbness and tingling, p. 74).

PAINFUL LEG

Most problems involving leg pain are the result of unaccustomed exercise having caused a sprain or strain to the muscles or ligaments. This type of pain will disappear when the leg is rested for a few days. However, persistent or severe pain or swelling should always be reported to your doctor

Severe pain following an injury, fall or violent movement

If the pain is severe, even when resting the leg, and/or there is a loss of movement, it's possible there is a fracture, or serious injury to the muscles or ligaments. Get to a hospital Accident and

Emergency Unit (casualty department) as soon as possible.

Treatment: The leg will probably be X-rayed. If there is a fracture you may need an operation to set the bone. A plaster cast or splint may be needed to support the leg while it heals.

Pain after strenuous exercise

A pulled muscle can result from unaccustomed or especially strenuous exercise.

Treatment: Rest the leg as much as possible until the pain has gone. A firm bandage to support the leg may help. When the pain has subsided, begin to exercise the leg again very gently to prevent stiffness. If there is swelling or the pain becomes worse or persists, see your doctor.

Sudden cramping pain in calf

Cramp is a sudden contraction of the muscle which makes it hard, tense and painful. It is usually brought on by exercise or by sitting or standing in an awkward position. Attacks of cramp, often at night, are especially common during pregnancy.

Treatment: Stretching the affected muscle can relieve the pain.

Straighten the affected leg, push your heel down firmly, and raise the toes up. The cramp should pass off in a few minutes. Doing this 'exercise' once or twice a day can help to prevent cramp.

Cramping pain in calf during exercise

Cramping pain that comes on during exercise and disappears with rest can be caused by poor circulation. During exercise the muscle needs more oxygen and an increased blood supply to carry it. Deposits of fatty material in the arteries can narrow them and reduce the blood flow. See your doctor.

Treatment: If your doctor suspects impaired circulation, he may refer you to hospital for tests. An angiogram and/or an ECG may be performed (see Medical diagnostic tests, pp. 300 and 304). A blood sample may be taken to measure the level of fats in the blood.

Following a low-fat diet, stopping smoking and taking regular exercise are all measures your doctor may recommend to reduce your risk of heart disease. In severe cases of blocked arteries, by-pass surgery may be considered.

Redness, swelling, tenderness or pain in a small area of the leg

An inflammation of part of a vein (thrombophlebitis), usually near the surface of the skin, can cause these symptoms. This may be the result of a minor injury to the vein, or as a complication of varicose veins. See your doctor.

Treatment: Your doctor may prescribe anti-inflammatory drugs to reduce swelling and antibiotics if any infection is present. A crêpe bandage can give support.

Painful, swollen calf, swollen ankles

A blood clot blocking the vein (deep vein thrombosis) can cause such symptoms. This can sometimes happen after injury or illness forces a long period of bed-rest. Smoking, obesity, varicose veins, diabetes and taking the contraceptive pill are some factors which can increase susceptibility to the formation of blood clots.

It is possible for blood clots to be carried to the heart and lungs with very serious results. See your doctor at once.

Treatment: If thrombosis is suspected, your doctor will refer you to hospital for tests such as angiography (see Medical diagnostic tests, p. 300) or venography (X-rays of blood vessels). Treatment may include drugs to prevent blood clotting further or to break down clots that have already formed.

Swollen blue veins in calves or insides of legs/ aching legs/swelling feet and ankles

These are symptoms of varicose veins. They are caused by a weakening of the valves in the walls of the veins that allows blood to collect and 'pool' there. A tendency to varicose veins is often inherited. Pregnancy and the hormonal changes of the menopause can also increase the risk of varicose veins. More women than men are affected.

Treatment: Self-help measures such as wearing support stockings or special bandages, avoiding standing for long periods, and resting with the legs up as often as possible are the only 'treatment' required by many sufferers. In severe cases, removing the veins or injecting a substance to 'block them off' may be recommended, and other veins then take over.

PAINFUL OR SWOLLEN JOINTS

The major joints of the body, the hips, knees and ankles, can sometimes be damaged by injury. Often the constant wear and tear they suffer gives rise to pain and stiffness that affect many people in later life.

Severe pain in a joint following a fall or injury

If you are unable to move the joint without severe pain and/or it looks misshapen, you may have dislocated it. Alternatively, damage to the bones, muscles or ligaments around it is a possibility.

Get to the casualty department of a hospital as soon as possible.

Treatment: You will probably be given X-rays to determine if the joint has been fractured. Surgery to re-position the joint may be needed. The joint may be plastered or put in a splint until it has healed.

One painful, red, swollen, very tender joint

Gout, caused by crystals of uric acid getting into the joint and giving intense irritation and pain, usually affects only one joint on a first attack. The base of the big toe is a common site, but gout can also attack the knee, ankle, wrist, foot or hand. Usually the attack subsides after two or three days.

However, gout can progressively affect more joints and cause almost continuous pain due to severe inflammation.

Treatment: Your doctor will probably arrange a blood test, and fluid may be taken from the affected joint to confirm the diagnosis. Anti-inflammatory drugs may be prescribed to control inflammation and pain. Drugs which reduce the levels of uric acid are suitable for some patients. Dietary changes, such as cutting down on excess alcohol and large, meaty meals, will usually be recommended.

Several painful, red, swollen, very tender joints

Rheumatoid arthritis is a serious joint disease. It is caused by the body's own immune system attacking the soft tissues of the joints and causing inflammation. The joints in the hands are commonly affected, but knees, shoulders and the neck can also be involved. See your doctor.

Treatment: Your doctor will probably arrange for a blood test and possibly X-rays of affected joints. Anti-inflammatory drugs and/or high doses of aspirin-like medicines may be prescribed.

Physiotherapy can help to keep the joint mobile. Joint replacement operations are very successful for patients disabled by arthritis.

Gradual pain and stiffness in one joint

Osteoarthritis (damage to the joint as a result of years of wear and tear) is very common in those over sixty. It is aggravated by injury or by years of over-use due to sport or repetitive occupational activities. The joint may swell and becomes painful with movement. See your doctor.

Treatment: Your doctor may arrange a blood test and/or X-rays of affected joints to confirm the diagnosis. Painkillers and/or anti-inflammatory drugs can relieve pain and swelling.

Physiotherapy helps to keep the joint mobile. Joint replacement operations can be very successful for those disabled by the disease.

Sudden pain and stiffness or swelling around one joint

Bursitis is an inflammation and swelling of the fluid-filled sac adjacent to a joint. It can be caused by prolonged kneeling (housemaid's knee), injury or over-use of the joint.

Treatment: The condition will usually clear up in a few days with rest. If inflammation or swelling persists consult your doctor.

He may prescribe anti-inflammatory drugs or in rare cases drain the fluid from the sac (the bursa).

Painful knee that sometimes seems to 'lock' or give way

A damaged cartilage can give these symptoms. This may be the result of a sports injury or a sudden strain or sprain. See your doctor.

Treatment: Cartilage damage is usually treated by surgery, often now undertaken through a tube (an arthroscope). Your doctor will probably refer you to a hospital specialist for diagnosis and treatment.

Stiffness and pain in shoulder, movement restricted

Frozen shoulder sometimes follows a minor injury, but it may develop for no apparent reason. It is caused by an inflammation of the lining of the shoulder joint and also, sometimes, by the muscles or ligament surrounding it. It can be intensely painful.

Treatment: Painkillers and/or ice-packs or heat treatment can ease the discomfort. It is important to keep the shoulder mobile by comfortably putting it through its usual movement range by using the other arm, or having someone else move it comfortably. Recovery is often slow. In severe cases your doctor may prescribe anti-inflammatory drugs, or an anti-inflammatory injection into the painful spot when there is one.

PALPITATIONS

Palpitations is a general term used to describe an unusually fast, strong, fluttering or rapid heartbeat. Exercise is the most common reason for the heart to beat harder or stronger than usual. However, feelings of anxiety, panic or fright can often cause such sensations, and so can alcohol, nicotine and caffeine.

If your heartbeat is often irregular or feels unusual when you are resting or in a calm mood, or if you also experience chest pain, dizziness or breathlessness, consult your doctor at once.

Palpitations with breathlessness, feeling faint, light-headed or dizzy

An abnormally fast heartbeat (tachycardia) can be caused by any of the circumstances outlined above – increased intake of tea, coffee or alcohol, excessive smoking, fear, fright or anxiety.

People who suffer panic attacks sometimes experience alarming changes in their heartbeat (see Anxiety, p. 27). However, these symptoms may also be a sign of a serious heart disorder and should be reported to your doctor straightaway.

Treatment: If your doctor suspects a heart disorder, he will arrange for you to have an electrocardiogram (see Medical diagnostic tests, p. 304) to check on your heart rhythms. Treatment will depend on any disorder found.

Palpitations with tiredness and/or weight loss/ increased appetite/diarrhoea/sweating

An over-active thyroid (thyrotoxicosis) can cause such symptoms.

See your doctor.

Treatment: If your doctor suspects an over-active thyroid, he will take blood tests to measure the level of thyroid hormones in the blood. You may be referred to hospital for a radioisotope scan of your thyroid. Treatment is with drugs or radioactive iodine to stop the over-production of thyroid hormones. In some cases, surgery to remove part of the thyroid gland is necessary.

Palpitations accompanied by feeling tired and weak/breathlessness when exercising/pallor

Anaemia, a condition in which there is too little haemoglobin in the blood, can cause these symptoms. Haemoglobin is a pigment which carries oxygen around the body. Low levels of it in the blood are usually the result of a shortage of iron in the diet. Pregnancy and heavy periods can often cause anaemia in women.

Treatment: Your doctor will take a blood sample to confirm anaemia. Anaemia due to iron shortage is treated with iron tablets or injection. Other causes of anaemia may need further investigation before treatment can be given.

RASH WITH FEVER

A rash or spots with a temperature of over 38° C (100° F) probably means the presence of one of the common childhood infectious illnesses (see p. 275), although with certain other symptoms meningitis is a possibility. This illness is a medical emergency and you should get help at once.

Raised, red, itchy spots on trunk and/or face that turn into blisters

Chickenpox can cause these symptoms, although it is rare in adults. One attack in childhood usually gives immunity for life.

The disease is caused by the virus which is also responsible for shingles in adults.

Chickenpox is usually a mild illness in children, but can be more severe in adults, sometimes causing complications such as breathing difficulties and pneumonia. Adults who have not had chickenpox should avoid contact with the illness. Women in the later stages of pregnancy should also take care to avoid it. Chickenpox may be serious in pregnancy, and can also infect a newborn baby.

Treatment: Take paracetamol or aspirin for fever and discomfort.

Drink plenty of fluids. Calamine lotion is soothing for the spots. Try not to scratch them as this can cause scars. If your temperature rises above 40° C (104° F), if you develop a bad cough or your eyes become painful, call your doctor. Recovery may take two or more weeks.

Spots or blotchy patches on head or neck with runny nose/cough/sore, red eyes/swollen glands

Measles, a highly contagious and potentially dangerous viral disease, causes these symptoms. In adults complications can include ear and chest infections. One attack in childhood usually gives lifelong immunity, but preferable, and strongly recommended, is the MMR vaccine which does so too, and which is now available for babies and children. This vaccine also protects against mumps and rubella – see below. Pregnant women should take great care to avoid measles if they did not have it as children. It can result in stillbirth.

Treatment: Take paracetamol or aspirin for fever and discomfort. Drink plenty of fluids. If you develop severe headache or earache, or if your cough gets worse, consult your doctor. He may prescribe antibiotics for any secondary infections.

Pink, spotty rash on face, trunk, arms and legs

German measles (rubella) can cause these symptoms. It may also give rise to a headache and swollen glands in the neck. German measles is usually a very mild illness in children. It can be slightly more of a nuisance to adults. It is serious only for pregnant women who have not had the illness in childhood, if caught during the first four months of pregnancy. The virus can cause blindness, deafness and heart defects in the fetus. Most women have a blood test early in pregnancy to check that they are immune to rubella.

Treatment: Aspirin or paracetamol can reduce fever. Otherwise, drink plenty of fluids, and rest if you feel unwell. Avoid contact with others, especially with any women who could be pregnant, for about a week.

Red, blotchy skin rash with vomiting/severe headache/stiff neck/dislike of strong light

Meningitis, an inflammation of the membranes covering the brain and spinal cord, causes these symptoms. This is a serious illness and you should get medical help at once.

Treatment: You will probably be admitted to hospital for a lumbar puncture (see Medical diagnostic tests, p. 306) to diagnose the illness. There are two types of meningitis. Bacterial meningitis is the more serious one. Treatment is by antibiotics, usually given by drip. Recovery may take several months.

Viral meningitis has no specific treatment, but you will be kept in hospital and will probably be given painkillers and fluids by drip. Recovery usually takes two to three weeks.

RINGING IN EARS

A condition known as tinnitus causes ringing, buzzing, whistling or hissing in one or both ears. The problem may be a symptom of a number of different disorders of the ear, and it usually occurs together with some loss of hearing (see Deafness, p. 45). Your doctor will usually arrange tests to discover if an underlying disorder is causing the noises, and this will be treated where possible.

In many cases there is very little that can be done to stop this symptom, which many sufferers find distressing. A radio, television or other source of noise can sometimes help to 'cover up' the ringing. Some sufferers find that a 'masking device' – headphones which play a random mixture of sounds – can help reduce the irritation of tinnitus.

RUNNY NOSE

A runny nose is most commonly a symptom of a cold. However, it can also be caused by allergies or by other viral infections.

Runny nose with sneezing and sore throat

These are sure signs of a cold. A cold is a viral infection that irritates the delicate mucous membrane lining the nose and throat, causing the nose to 'run'. The nasal discharge is usually clear and watery at first, but may become thicker and opaque as the cold progresses. If the discharge turns yellowish or green, it is usually a sign that a secondary infection has become established.

Treatment: Stay at home in a warm room and drink plenty of clear fluids like fruit juices. Aspirin or paracetamol can reduce feverish symptoms. Inhaling warm steam from a basin gives relief from a 'blocked up' nose. If nasal discharge is still severe after ten days, or if the cold seems to have affected your ears or chest, see your doctor. He may prescribe antibiotics if there is any secondary infection.

Runny nose with sneezing or sore eyes

Irritation from smoke or other fumes can cause such symptoms.

Alternatively, an allergy to pollen, house dust, house dust mites, animal hair or other irritants (hay fever, allergic rhinitis) could be the problem.

Treatment: If fumes are causing the problem, the symptoms should subside once the irritant has disappeared. For other allergies try, if possible, to discover the cause of the symptoms and avoid it where practical. In severe cases, consult your doctor. He may prescribe anti-histamine tablets or other forms of treatment to reduce symptoms. Allergy tests can be undertaken to try to discover the source of the allergic reaction, but these are not always successful.

Thick nasal discharge and pain in face with/ following a cold

Sinusitis, an inflammation of the sinuses in the face, can cause these symptoms (see Pain in face, p. 78).

SKIN PROBLEMS

Infections, inflammation and many other types of disorder can affect the skin (see also Moles and warts, p. 71, and Spots and rashes, p. 105). Any open sores that do not heal within three weeks, changes in appearance of long-standing moles or warts, new areas of pigmentation, or slow-growing lumps, should always be reported to your doctor because of the possibility of skin cancer.

Patches of inflamed, itchy skin

Eczema or dermatitis are possible causes of inflamed, itchy or sore skin patches. There are several forms of eczema and dermatitis:

Atopic or infantile eczema

This is an allergic skin rash that often starts in babies or young children. It has a tendency to run in families. Children who suffer from this type of eczema may also be prone to hay fever or other allergies. The rash usually begins on the wrists, the inside of the elbows or the backs of knees, but may spread further. It can be intensely itchy and can become weepy and infected when children scratch. See your doctor.

Treatment: Avoiding soaps and using instead creams to cleanse and soothe the skin will help. In severe cases, steroid ointments to reduce inflammation and antibiotics for infection are prescribed.

Wearing only cotton clothes next to the skin and avoiding harsh detergents is usually recommended. Children do tend to 'grow out' of this problem as they reach adolescence.

Contact or irritant eczema

This often affects the hands, and is caused by direct contact with an irritating substance, for example harsh chemicals or detergents. Certain metals in jewellery, perfumes or chemicals in cosmetics, as well as some plants, can cause the condition. It can produce a dry, itchy rash and flaky skin or blistering and soreness.

Treatment: Avoid the irritant substance if known. Wear protective gloves and use plenty of moisturizer if the rash affects the hands. Mild steroid creams to reduce inflammation can be bought from the chemist's. If self-help measures do not improve the condition within a few days, see your doctor. He may prescribe a different kind of steroid cream.

Seborrhoeic dermatitis

This is a red, scaly, itchy rash that develops on the face, especially on the nose and eyebrows. It can also affect the chest and back and the scalp, where it causes a severe form of dandruff.

The exact cause is not known.

Treatment: Avoid scratching affected areas or exposing them to irritating substances. Consult your doctor if the rash is extensive or worrying. He may prescribe a steroid cream or ointment, or suggest other measures.

Blackheads, raised spots with white centres, painful red lumps under the skin affecting face, chest and back

Acne is a general term used to describe these types of skin disorder. It occurs when hair follicles become blocked by excess production of oils in the skin.

Treatment: Thorough washing of the affected areas twice a day is recommended. There are many lotions and washes that can be bought at the chemist's that aim to reduce the possibility of infection. Other products have a mild abrasive action to remove dead skin cells that can block pores. It is usually recommended that the treatment, to be effective, be maintained for at least three months. If acne continues to be unsightly or embarrassing, see your doctor. A long-term course of low-dose antibiotics can often help clear the condition. Occasionally, referral to a skin specialist will be advised.

Sore blisters around the mouth

Cold sores are caused by the virus herpes simplex which most people have in their bodies. This can become activated by a cold or other infection, or by strong sunlight. Some people are especially prone to bouts of cold sores when they are run-down, and women around the time of their period.

Treatment: Soothing ointments can be bought at the chemist's which may speed healing. For persistent or troublesome outbreaks, your doctor may be able to prescribe an antiviral ointment.

Patches of inflamed red skin covered by white, flaky scales, often on elbows, knees or scalp

Psoriasis is a common skin disorder causing such symptoms. The exact cause is not known, but it tends to run in families. In severe cases, outbreaks of the skin problem may be accompanied by painful swelling and stiffness in the joints. See your doctor.

Treatment: Your doctor can prescribe several soothing ointments or creams which can help. Drug treatment and/or phototherapy (treatment with ultraviolet light) can also help.

One or more open, painful sores on skin

Skin ulcers can occur after injury or infection. On the legs, they are often the result of poor circulation caused by diabetes or a circulation problem.

Treatment: Keep the sore clean and dry. Protect with a bandage or light dressing if necessary. If the ulcer does not heal within three weeks, or if more break out, see your doctor.

Flushing with very red nose and cheeks

Rosacea is quite common in middle age and affects women more than men. The disorder may also cause acne-like lumps on the skin.

Flushing may be brought on by hot rooms, alcohol, coffee or spicy foods. See your doctor if the condition causes embarrassment.

Treatment: A course of antibiotics may help the condition of your skin, although often the problem does recur. In many people it disappears of its own accord after a few years.

SLEEP PROBLEMS

As many as one in three adults have trouble sleeping at some time in their lives. They may have problems falling asleep at night, wake in the night and be unable to sleep again, or find that they wake very early in the morning. Lack of sleep can cause irritability, feelings of tiredness, or fears of not being able to cope during the day. Many insomniacs worry that not getting enough sleep will damage their health. However, studies show that lack of sleep is not as harmful as people think.

The real test of whether you are getting enough sleep or not is if you feel extremely sleepy during the day. Feeling sleepy must not be confused, though, with the feelings of lethargy or disinterest that can be a feature of depression. Depressed people often say they are 'tired' because they can't sleep when, in fact, it is their depression, not lack of sleep, that is causing the problem.

Depression and anxiety are two of the most common reasons for sleep disturbance (see Anxiety, p. 27, and Depression, p. 47).

Difficulty sleeping is also common during pregnancy, particularly in the later months (see Tiredness and insomnia, p. 199). As we age, we need less sleep, so if you are over sixty it is quite normal for you not to need as much sleep as you did when you were younger.

Trouble falling asleep at night

Persistent anxieties (see Anxiety, p. 27) that cause worry at bedtime can prevent sleep. Generally, sleep patterns return to normal once the difficulty has been resolved.

The caffeine in tea, coffee, cola and cocoa stimulates the central nervous system and can make it difficult for you to sleep if you've drunk too much of any of these during the day. Likewise, a heavy meal before bedtime, or drinking too much alcohol, can cause sleeplessness.

Try these self-help measures to avoid sleeplessness and get a good night's rest:

- Try not to worry about lack of sleep. Worry itself causes sleeplessness, and it's very unlikely that lack of sleep will do your health any harm
- Don't go to bed until you feel sleepy, however late this is. If you get to bed and cannot go to sleep within fifteen minutes, then get up, leave the bedroom, and do something to occupy yourself until you feel sleepy. It's important to associate bed with sleep, not with tossing and turning
- Avoid daytime naps. They will make you feel less tired at night
- Avoid tea, coffee or heavy drinking before bedtime. A warm, milky drink or a small tot of alcohol may make you feel sleepy
- Try to take some exercise during the day to tire you physically
- Make your bedroom comfortable. Ensure that it is not too hot or cold; eliminate any irritating noises or light
- A warm bath before bedtime can be relaxing
- Set an alarm clock to make sure that you get up at the same time each morning. Don't be tempted to sleep in for a couple of hours at the weekend or if you've had a bad night, as this will disrupt your sleep patterns
- Learn a few simple relaxation exercises such as deep breathing

or relaxing all of the body's muscles. Practise them before you try to sleep

Waking early in the morning

Waking early can begin to occur once we age and need less sleep.

It is no cause for concern. Early waking, especially if you brood over problems at this time, can also be a symptom of depression (see Depression, p. 47).

Sleep problems after stopping sleeping-tablets or tranquillizers

Sleeping-pills work by reducing the activity of the brain to allow sleep. Ideally, they should be taken only for a few weeks at a time during particularly difficult periods, such as after a bereavement. However, many people who have taken them for much longer periods find that they experience withdrawal symptoms and have trouble sleeping when they try to stop.

Treatment: Follow the advice outlined above for helping you get to sleep. Try to resist asking for more pills once you have decided to stop. If sleeping problems continue for more than a month, seek your doctor's help. He may be able to put you in touch with a self-help group or a counsellor who can assist you through this difficult period.

SORE MOUTH OR TONGUE

There are several minor conditions which can give rise to sore areas on the lips, mouth or tongue. Usually, these are no cause for concern and will heal naturally. However, if soreness or pain persist for several weeks, or if sore areas will not heal, consult your doctor. In rare cases, such problems can be a sign of mouth cancer.

Very painful inflamed spots inside mouth or lips or on tongue

Mouth ulcers look like little white craters and can be very sore indeed. They are caused by breaks in the mucous membrane that lines the mouth. Usually, they will heal within a few days and don't need any special treatment. Rinsing the mouth with an antiseptic mouthwash or with warm salty water can help relieve pain and speed healing. Ointments and lozenges that do the same thing can be bought from the chemist's. If ulcers don't heal within three weeks, or if they recur, see your doctor.

Sore tongue

A red, painful and sore tongue (glossitis) can be caused by a number of different disorders including anaemia, vitamin deficiency, or infection with the herpes simplex virus that causes cold sores. Burning the tongue with a hot drink, inadvertently biting the tongue, excess smoking and/or drinking, too much spicy food, or irritation by badly fitting dentures or sharp teeth, can also cause this problem. See your doctor.

Treatment: Your doctor will try to discover the cause of the soreness and will treat you accordingly. Avoid acidic or spicy foods that aggravate the soreness. Rinsing regularly with a mouthwash can help.

Sore, creamy yellow areas on tongue or in mouth

Oral thrush, which is a fungal infection, is a possibility. See your doctor.

Treatment: Your doctor may take a sample of the yellow creamy discharge to confirm his diagnosis. Treatment for thrush is with a course of anti-fungal tablets.

Painful, swollen or bleeding gums

An inflammation of the gums (gingivitis) is usually caused by not paying enough attention to oral hygiene. See your dentist.

Treatment: Your dentist will thoroughly clean your teeth and remove any hard deposits that have accumulated. He will show you how to clean your teeth thoroughly yourself and how to use dental floss to remove the plaque that causes gum disease. Proper cleaning and six-monthly visits to the dentist should stop the problem recurring.

Blisters or sores on or around the lips

Cold sores are probably the cause of these (see Skin problems, p. 95).

SORE OR PAINFUL EYES

Infection or inflammation are the most usual reason for sore or painful eye(s).

Pain or soreness due to something in eye

Specks of dirt or eyelashes can be dislodged very gently using the moistened corner of a clean handkerchief. If the particle cannot be seen, it may be on the inside of the eyelid, which can be gently folded back. If the foreign body cannot be removed like this seek your doctor's help. Never try to remove an object embedded in the eyeball, a chip of metal or a particle over the iris, yourself.

White of eye bloodshot/sticky discharge from eye

An inflammation of the membrane covering the eye (conjunctivitis) is the most likely cause. Conjunctivitis is very common. It
is often caused by infection from cold, flu or other germs. See
your doctor.

Treatment: Your doctor will prescribe antibiotic drops or ointment. Wipe any sticky discharge from the eye using cotton wool
dipped in cooled boiled water. Use each piece only once to avoid
spreading the infection, and use a separate piece for the other
eye. Avoid sharing face-flannels or towels with other family
members for the same reason.

Red, itchy eyelids

Inflammation of the eyelid (blepharitis) can cause sore, scaly skin.
Sometimes this can be related to dandruff. See your doctor.

Treatment: Your doctor will probably prescribe a bicarbonate of
soda lotion or an ointment that will clear up the condition.

Sore, red lump on eyelid

A stye is a boil-like infection that forms at the base of an eyelash.
Generally, a stye will either dry up of its own accord or burst
within a week. It needs no special treatment other than wiping
away any sticky discharge with a clean piece of moistened cotton
wool. If the stye doesn't heal, if the eye becomes red or painful,
or if you often suffer from styes, see your doctor.

Treatment: Your doctor may prescribe an antibiotic ointment or
drops for the stye. He may ask about your general health and
well-being and suggest measures to improve them if you are
run-down and often suffer from styes.

Aching pain in and above eye/foggy or blurred vision and/or seeing haloes around lights

Acute glaucoma, a serious condition in which too much fluid in the eyeball causes pressure to build up, is possible, especially if you are over forty. Seek medical help urgently.

Treatment: You will probably be referred to a hospital specialist right away. Treatment is with eyedrops and other drugs to reduce pressure in the eyeball as quickly as possible. Once the pressure is controlled, surgery may be necessary to prevent the problem recurring.

Watering eyes

Chemical fumes or an allergic reaction to something can cause the eyes to water and become sore. There is no specific treatment for this other than avoiding the source of the irritation if it is known.

Sore, painful eyes that don't water

A number of uncommon disorders of the auto-immune system can lead to not enough fluid being produced in the tear ducts. As a result, the eyes feel dry, gritty and painful. See your doctor.

Treatment: Your doctor will probably take steps to investigate the cause of the problem. He will prescribe special eyedrops, which act as artificial tears, to be used frequently.

SORE THROAT

A sore throat is a very common symptom. It is most often the first sign of a cold, and usually disappears as the cold gets better. Taking plenty of cold drinks and gargling with soluble aspirin or paracetamol can relieve the painful effects of a sore throat.

Sore throat with high temperature/cough/ headache/aches and pains

A viral infection such as flu is the most likely cause of these symptoms.

Treatment: Stay in bed and take aspirin or paracetamol for the fever and discomfort. If you are no better within two days, or if other symptoms such as a rash or breathlessness develop, see your doctor.

Sore throat with tenderness and swelling under jaw

If you have not had the illness in childhood, mumps (see Common childhood infectious illnesses, p. 275) is a possibility. This viral infection causes the salivary and other glands to swell, and in men can also affect the testicles. Occasionally, it can lead to infertility. Call your doctor.

Treatment: You may need to rest in bed for several days. Your doctor will advise drinking plenty of fluids and taking aspirin or paracetamol to reduce fever and pain. Sometimes anti-inflammatory drugs are prescribed if the testicles are painfully inflamed and swollen.

Sore throat/pain on swallowing/earache/ swollen glands in neck

Tonsillitis or pharyngitis (inflammation of the throat) can cause these symptoms. These inflammations are caused by infection with a virus or bacteria, and often follow a cold or flu.

Treatment: Rest, drinking plenty of fluids, and taking aspirin or paracetamol to reduce pain are usually all the treatment that's needed. Avoid smoking or drinking alcohol, which can aggravate the throat and tonsils. Generally, the symptoms should subside within two days or so. If the pain persists, or if the infection seems to spread further, consult your doctor.

Sore throat with loss of voice

See Hoarseness, p. 68.

SPEECH PROBLEMS

There are several disorders which may affect speech. Difficulty or slowness in finding and using the right words can be due to a disturbance or disorder of the centres in the brain which control language. The side-effects of certain drugs can sometimes cause speech problems. If you are taking any medicines, and your speech becomes slowed or slurred, see your doctor about it. A disorder of the mouth, face or tongue can also cause difficulty in forming or pronouncing words.

Difficulty speaking accompanied by dizziness/ weakness in arms or legs/disturbed vision/ confusion or forgetfulness

A stroke or a transient ischaemic attack can cause such symptoms (see Confusion and forgetfulness, p. 39).

Stammering or stuttering

Repeated hesitation or delay in saying what you want, difficulty in pronouncing words, or the repetition of certain sounds, usually begins in childhood. The cause of stuttering is not really known.

Some doctors believe it is due to anxiety; others that it is the result of some form of subtle brain damage.

Treatment: Stammering can often be improved with the help of a specialist speech therapist. There are many techniques which can improve fluency and confidence in speech.

SPOTS AND RASHES

Spots and rashes are not usually serious, but they may be signs of several different types of disorder. With a raised temperature, they usually indicate one of the childhood infectious illnesses such as measles or chickenpox (see Rash with fever, p. 89). Inflamed or itchy rashes can be caused by skin problems such as eczema or dermatitis (see Skin problems, p. 93), or by allergic reactions or infections. Occasionally, other types of rash may indicate a more serious type of underlying disorder.

Painful, blistery rash on one side of body

Shingles, a viral infection of the nerves to the skin, could be a possibility, especially if you are over fifty. See your doctor at once, as prompt treatment can limit the severity of the illness.

Treatment: If shingles is in its early stages, the doctor may prescribe an antiviral drug. Otherwise, an ointment and/or painkillers may be offered. The blisters associated with the illness should clear within three weeks. Unfortunately, pain from damage to the nerve endings may persist for weeks or even, in a few cases, months.

Itchy, raised patches with white or yellowish middle, redness around outside

Nettle rash or hives (urticaria) can cause this type of rash. It can be due to an allergic reaction to certain foods, drugs or chemicals, but often the cause isn't known. Occasionally, there may also be swelling of another part of the body. If the face or mouth swells, this can be dangerous. See your doctor at once.

Treatment: Such rashes usually subside after a few hours. Calamine lotion, cold compresses or anti-histamine cream or tablets from the chemist's can relieve itching. If you have repeated or persistent attacks, see your doctor. He may be able to treat the problem with anti-inflammatory drugs.

Round patches of red skin with scaly surface

A fungal infection such as ringworm can cause this type of rash (see p. 262).

Several raised, very itchy spots

Insect or flea bites can cause such spots.

Treatment: Calamine lotion or anti-histamine cream can relieve itching. Try not to scratch the spot; it may become infected.

Check your cat or dog for fleas and treat if necessary. Inspect any possible sources of fleas or bed-bugs in the home and take steps to deal with any problem found.

Very itchy, reddish lumps on chest, arms and legs/grey lines or red spots between fingers and on wrists

Scabies, an infection inflicted by a skin parasite, causes such symptoms.

See your doctor.

Treatment: Your doctor will prescribe an insecticide lotion if he finds scabies. He will advise everyone else in the household to be treated at the same time, since scabies is very contagious.

Purplish or reddish-brown areas of spots

This type of rash (purpura) can be caused by bleeding under the skin. There can be many causes. In elderly people, thinning tissues result in blood vessels being easily injured or ruptured.

Inflammation of the blood vessels, often due to an allergic reaction to food or a drug, can cause bleeding. Certain blood disorders including anaemia and leukaemia, infections, and other 'chemical' disorders of the body can also cause bleeding beneath the skin. See your doctor straightaway if you develop this type of rash.

Treatment: Your doctor may need to do a blood test or arrange for other types of test to be undertaken in hospital to discover the cause of the rash. Treatment will depend on the diagnosis.

STIFF NECK

Stiff neck is a very common symptom and usually comes on suddenly for no apparent reason. Often it is noticed first thing on waking in the morning. It is usually due to a spasm of the muscles at the side or the back of the neck, and this will pass naturally within a day or two. If you have persistent or severe pain or stiffness you should see your doctor.

Stiff neck following sudden or violent jolt

A whiplash injury can strain the muscles and ligaments in the neck and cause pain. If the pain is no better within a day, see your doctor.

Treatment: Your doctor will advise you to rest as much as possible, and may recommend that you wear a supportive collar until the injury has healed.

Severe pain and/or shooting pain down arm/arm feels weak

A prolapsed (slipped) disc in the neck can cause severe pain. This occurs when part of the pulpy centre of the disc that separates each vertebra protrudes and presses on the spinal nerve. It can happen suddenly as a result of injury, but usually is a more gradual process caused by wear and tear. See your doctor.

Treatment: Your doctor will probably arrange an X-ray of the back and possibly other tests to confirm the diagnosis. He may advise resting flat in bed, wearing a surgical collar and/or heat treatment, physiotherapy or other treatments once the pain has subsided.

Stiffness and pain gradually getting worse over a few months

Arthritis of the bones in the neck caused by wear and tear (cervical spondylitis) is possible, especially if you are over fifty. See your doctor.

Treatment: Your doctor may arrange for an X-ray to confirm the diagnosis. Treatment aims to reduce pain and rest the neck, possibly with a surgical collar at first. When the pain has lessened, physiotherapy, massage and exercises to keep the joints as mobile as possible are usually suggested. If pain is caused by pressure on the spinal nerve, an operation to correct this is sometimes possible.

Painful or stiff neck with severe headache/ nausea or vomiting/drowsiness or confusion/dislike of bright lights

Meningitis, a dangerous inflammation of the membranes around the brain and the central nervous system, is possible (see Rash with fever, p. 90). Get medical help at once.

SWALLOWING DIFFICULTY

A sore throat is the most usual reason for a problem with swallowing. However, pain or difficulty in swallowing that is not caused by a sore throat or other simple explanation can occasionally be a sign of a more serious disorder and should be reported to your doctor.

Trouble swallowing/painful throat

It is possible that a piece of food, a fish-bone for example, may have become lodged in your throat and be causing soreness. See your doctor.

Treatment: Your doctor may be able to locate and remove any particle by examining you. Failing this, an X-ray may be necessary to pinpoint the source of the trouble so that it can be removed.

Trouble swallowing/food seems to stick in throat/pain in chest/burning sensation

Hiatus hernia, a condition where part of the stomach protrudes upwards through the chest wall leaking acid juices into the windpipe, can cause heartburn and wind and make swallowing seem difficult. It can be made worse by lying down or bending over. See your doctor.

Treatment: Your doctor will advise taking small, frequent meals and avoiding alcohol and tobacco, which both irritate stomach complaints. He may also advise losing weight if you are too heavy. Antacid medicines can help relieve symptoms. In severe cases an operation to correct the problem can be performed.

Trouble swallowing because of dry mouth

Insufficient production of saliva is usually a temporary condition. It can sometimes be caused by fear or anxiety. Certain drugs may also have this effect. Occasionally, an infection of the salivary glands may cause them to make less saliva than normal. A rare condition called Sjogren's syndrome can also cause a dry mouth. See your doctor if the problem persists or is troublesome.

Treatment: Your doctor will try to discover the cause of the problem and treat it accordingly.

Trouble swallowing/unexplained weight loss of more than 10 lbs (4.5 kg) in last ten weeks

A growth in the throat is a slight possibility. See your doctor.

Treatment: Your doctor will arrange for you to have tests such as a barium X-ray or endoscopy (see Medical diagnostic tests, pp. 300 and 304) in hospital. Treatment will depend on the cause of the problem.

SWEATING PROFUSELY

Sweating is the body's natural defence against becoming too hot.

As sweat on the skin evaporates, it cools and reduces body temperature. Some people naturally sweat more than others, and this is no cause for concern. However, sweating that is not caused by exercise or by being too hot, or sweating far more than is normal for you, can be a sign of a number of disorders.

Sweating and obesity

Carrying a great deal of excess weight can put such a strain on your body that even everyday activities seem like exercise.

Consult the Ideal weight charts on page 313. If you are over-weight, you should make a serious effort to slim down. See your doctor if you feel you need help or advice with this.

Sweating with tiredness and/or unexplained weight loss/trembling/increased appetite/palpitations

An over-active thyroid (thyrotoxicosis) can cause such symptoms.

See your doctor.

Treatment: If your doctor suspects an over-active thyroid, he will take blood tests to measure the level of thyroid hormones in the blood. You may be referred to hospital for a radioisotope scan of your thyroid. Treatment is with drugs or a radioactive medicine to stop the over-production of thyroid hormones. In some cases, surgery to remove part of the thyroid gland is necessary.

Sweating at night with weight loss/persistent cough

Tuberculosis (TB), an infection of the lungs, can cause these symptoms. See your doctor.

Treatment: Your doctor will arrange for you to have a chest X-ray and samples of phlegm and blood will be taken for analysis.

If tuberculosis is diagnosed, you will be treated with a long course of antibiotics taken over several months.

Sweating at night just before or during a period

Changes in the hormone balance cause increased sweating in some women around the time of a period. This is no cause for concern.

Sweats and hot flushes in women approaching the menopause

If you are over forty-five and your periods have started to become irregular, the change of life could be causing these symptoms.

They are no cause for concern and should pass in a year or so.

However, if the symptom is troublesome, see your doctor. He may prescribe hormone replacement therapy (HRT), which can control these symptoms.

Sweating when anxious or excited

Stress can cause an increase in sweating and this in itself is no cause for concern. However, if serious emotional stress or anxiety is causing excessive sweating, see your doctor. He may be able to suggest some ways to help deal with the underlying problem.

Sweating after drinking alcohol or taking large doses of aspirin

Both these drugs can cause increased sweating. If alcohol regularly causes this problem you should make an effort to cut down your consumption. See your doctor if you need to take large doses of aspirin to control pain. He may be able to suggest other ways of helping with the problem.

SWOLLEN ABDOMEN

A problem with the digestive organs or, if you are a woman, with the reproductive organs, can cause abdominal swelling. Some causes of abdominal swelling are harmless – wind, for example.

However, if the swelling is also painful, the cause may be more serious and you should get medical help at once.

Are you due to have a period/ could you be pregnant?

Fluid retention just before a period can cause abdominal swelling. This is no cause for concern in itself, but if the problem bothers you, or if you suffer other symptoms such as mood swings or irritability, see your doctor. He may be able to prescribe drugs to reduce fluid retention or to help other symptoms.

A pregnancy will begin to show signs of abdominal swelling from about the twelfth week. If you think you could be pregnant, see your doctor.

Sudden abdominal swelling with pain and/or vomiting

An obstruction of the intestine is possible. This is a medical emergency and you should get help at once.

Treatment: If an intestinal obstruction is suspected, you will probably be admitted to hospital for a thorough abdominal examination which may include an X-ray or ultrasound scan (see Medical diagnostic tests, p. 308). Surgery to deal with any blockage may be necessary.

Long-standing abdominal pain with puffy or swollen ankles and/or passing less urine than normal

Fluid retention as a result of a heart, liver or kidney problem is possible. See your doctor.

Treatment: Your doctor will arrange for you to have the tests appropriate to the condition he suspects. Treatment will depend on the underlying cause of the symptoms.

Swelling reduces slightly on passing urine

Retention of urine in the bladder can cause such symptoms. In men, this may be due to an enlarged prostate gland. See your doctor at once.

Treatment: Your doctor will examine you and arrange appropriate tests in hospital if necessary. Intravenous pyelography (see Medical diagnostic tests, p. 306) will probably be performed and blood and urine samples will be taken. In severe cases of enlarged prostate, surgery to remove the gland is usually recommended.

TIREDNESS

Feeling tired all the time or lacking energy is a very common symptom. It can be due to something as simple as not getting enough sleep or working too hard, or it may be a sign of a more serious disorder that needs investigation by your doctor.

Feeling tired with missed period

Overwhelming tiredness is a common symptom of early pregnancy. If you are suddenly very tired and have also missed a period, arrange to have a pregnancy test if it is possible that you may have conceived.

Tiredness with feeling low in spirits and/or lack of interest in things/difficulty concentrating or making decisions/frequent headaches

Depression can make you feel tired and unwell (see Depression, p. 47).

Feeling tired due to lack of sleep or disturbed sleep

See Sleep problems, p. 96.

Tiredness accompanied by feeling cold more than normal and/or unusual weight gain/ thin or brittle hair/dry skin

These can be symptoms of hypothyroidism, a condition in which the thyroid gland fails to produce enough hormone. This problem is most common in middle-aged women. See your doctor.

Treatment: Your doctor may take tests to diagnose the condition, or he may send you to a hospital specialist. Treatment for under-active thyroid is with tablets of thyroxine to replace the natural hormone the body is failing to produce. The tablets need to be taken for life in the same way that diabetic sufferers need to take insulin every day. Most patients feel much better soon after treatment begins, and return to normal within a few weeks.

Tiredness accompanied by feeling faint or weak and/or breathlessness/pallor/palpitations

Anaemia, a disorder in which there is too little of the pigment haemoglobin in the blood, is possible. This disorder is most often due to insufficient iron in the diet. It can affect women who have heavy periods, and is common during pregnancy when there are extra demands on the body for iron. See your doctor.

Treatment: Your doctor will take a blood test. If your iron levels are low, he will prescribe iron in the form of tablets or injections. He will also advise improving your diet to include plenty of iron-rich foods such as meat, spinach and lentils.

Other forms of anaemia not due to iron deficiency need further investigation before they can be treated.

Tiredness and extreme muscle weakness and/or muscular pain/ headache/dizziness/nausea/ inability to concentrate/depression/sleep disturbance following a viral infection such as flu, cold or other illness

This group of symptoms is typical of a disorder known as myalgic encephalomyelitis (ME), sometimes called post-viral fatigue syndrome and, in the past, 'yuppie flu'. The cause of ME is not yet known and is the subject of much medical debate. Possible explanations for the condition include a persistent viral infection or damage to the immune system following a viral infection. There is no diagnostic test for ME, although sufferers often show evidence of a current or recent viral infection. The condition usually clears up in time, although some people suffer recurring bouts of illness over a number of years.

Treatment: Because the cause is as yet unknown, there is no specific medical treatment for ME. Doctors normally advise rest and then taking exercise as soon as the patient is well enough.

Many sufferers try self-help measures such as careful diet, avoiding alcohol and caffeine, and alternative therapies.

Psychotherapy is helpful for some patients who suffer depression associated with ME.

Tiredness after drinking alcohol

Drinking even moderate amounts of alcohol regularly can have a depressant effect and make you feel tired.

Treatment: Make a serious effort to reduce your alcohol intake to recommended limits – 14 units per week for women, that is 14 pub measures of spirits or 14 pub-measure glasses of wine, or 14 half- pints of beer, and 21 units per week for men, that is 21 pub measures of spirits, 21 pub-measure glasses of wine, or 21 half-pints of beer. If you have difficulty cutting down on drinking, see your doctor for help.

TOOTHACHE

Toothache is nearly always caused by dental decay. Decay occurs when sugars in the food we eat are converted to acids by bacteria in the mouth. These acids soon attack the tooth enamel. When decay reaches the point where it is detected by the very sensitive nerve at the centre of each tooth, the result can be very painful.

Thoroughly brushing your teeth at least once a day and using dental floss to dislodge any persistent debris is the best insurance against toothache and tooth decay. You should see your dentist every six months, or as advised, for a check-up and for attention to any problems that have developed.

Toothache when eating very hot, cold or sweet foods

The early stages of tooth decay, or a leaking or cracked filling, can cause such pain. See your dentist.

Treatment: The dentist will remove the filling and/or decay and fill the tooth. He may take X-rays to check for problems in any other teeth. If the pain was caused by tooth decay, he will explain how to clean your teeth properly to avoid such problems in future.

Throbbing or stabbing pain in tooth/ very painful to bite or chew on

Advanced dental decay or an abscess in or around the tooth resulting from infection are possible. See your dentist.

Treatment: Your dentist will examine your mouth and may take X-rays. He will remove any decay or inadequate filling. An abscess will need to be drained. Root canal work to remove decayed tissue from inside the tooth will probably be needed.

Antibiotics may be required if infection from an abscess has spread beyond the tooth.

In some cases the tooth may need to be removed, but this is avoided where at all possible.

Toothache after a filling

It is quite normal to have some extra sensitivity after a tooth has been filled. The pain may be sharp, but usually it will only last for a few seconds at a time. Occasionally a filling may be too 'high' or uneven and may be uncomfortable when you bite on it. If such problems persist for more than a few days after a filling, return to your dentist who will take steps to remedy the problem.

Sensitivity to hot or cold

Sharp pain as a result of very hot or cold liquids or foods can sometimes be a sign of tooth decay. It may also be a result of the gum margins around some teeth receding and exposing sensitive tooth enamel. This can happen as a result of gum disease or bad brushing technique. See your dentist.

Treatment: Your dentist will examine you and try to discover the cause of the problem. If poor dental hygiene or bad brushing are to blame, he may refer you to a hygienist for thorough cleaning and instruction on the best way to care for your teeth. Many dentists now refer routinely.

TWITCHING AND TREMBLING

Occasional twitching or trembling movements affect almost everyone from time to time. They may often be brought on by anxiety or tiredness. A slight persistent tremor not caused by illness is also common in elderly people. In some people, a tendency to tremble is inherited and is no cause for concern.

Certain drugs, including those used to treat depression, can cause trembling. If you have recently been prescribed medication and find you suffer this side-effect, or if trying to give up or cut down on medication such as tranquillizers causes such a problem, seek your doctor's help. Drinking a great deal of coffee can cause shaking in some people. The problem usually disappears if intake is reduced or stopped. In some cases, twitching or trembling can be a sign of a disorder that needs investigation by your doctor.

Trembling or shaking movements of the hands or arms, worse when the hand or arm is at rest

Parkinson's disease, an illness which affects the nerves controlling movement, can cause such symptoms. This illness mostly affects people over the age of fifty-five; it is uncommon in younger people. See your doctor.

Treatment: No treatment is usually necessary in mild cases of Parkinson's disease. If the trembling becomes worse, drugs may be prescribed to help control it. Your doctor will be able to put you in touch with organizations which help and support sufferers from this illness.

Trembling with excessive sweating and/or tiredness/unexplained weight loss/palpitations

An over-active thyroid gland (thyrotoxicosis) can cause such symptoms (see Palpitations, p. 88).

Trembling after cutting down on drinking alcohol

If you are regularly a heavy drinker, and have recently cut down, shaking can be among the withdrawal symptoms. This indicates that you have become dependent on alcohol and that you need to continue to drink less or to stop drinking altogether. See your doctor for help with this.

Treatment: Your doctor may be able to prescribe a drug to help with the symptoms of withdrawal from alcohol. He will also be able to put you in touch with a support group for those who want to give up drink.

URINARY PROBLEMS

If you suddenly find that you need to pass much more, or much less, urine a day than normal, you should see your doctor at once.

Trouble beginning or controlling the flow of urine should also be reported to him. If you are suddenly unable to pass urine, you should seek medical help at once. It's possible that the urethra could be blocked, and damage to the bladder or kidneys can result if you don't get prompt treatment. If you have pain when passing urine, or if you 'leak' urine, see Men's symptoms, p. 145, or Women's symptoms, p. 153.

Passing large amounts of urine with tiredness and/or weight loss/hunger/great thirst

Such symptoms can be caused by diabetes mellitus (sugar diabetes). This is a disorder that results from the pancreas not producing enough of the hormone insulin. Insulin enables the body to convert food into energy. See your doctor.

Treatment: Your doctor will probably ask for a urine sample. If he suspects diabetes, he will ask you to return for a blood test later. Diabetes can be controlled with diet alone in some people, and in others, diet plus tablets. Others need regular daily injections of insulin to replace what the body should be producing.

All diabetics must pay careful attention to what they eat, and are instructed thoroughly on diet at specialist diabetic clinics.

Passing much more, or much less, urine than normal

It's possible that you could have a kidney problem. See your doctor at once.

Treatment: If your doctor suspects kidney trouble, he will probably take urine and blood samples. He may refer you straightaway for intravenous pyelography, a special X-ray of the kidneys, or for ultrasound scanning (see Medical diagnostic tests, pp. 306 and 308) or other tests. Treatment will depend on the result of these tests.

Passing small amounts of urine and/or a very weak stream/urine flow slow in starting

It's possible that a narrowing of the urethra (the tube that carries urine away from the bladder) may cause these symptoms. In women, this can sometimes be caused by a difficult childbirth or by infection (see Bladder control, poor, p. 153). In older men, the problem is sometimes the result of an enlarged prostate gland (see Painful urination, p. 145).

VISION PROBLEMS

Any difficulties or changes in your vision such as blurring, seeing double, spots, flashing lights or loss of sight should be brought to your doctor's attention immediately. Such problems need to be diagnosed and, when necessary, treated promptly in order to avoid the possibility of damage that could threaten your sight.

Sudden loss of all, or part, of vision in one or both eyes

This is a medical emergency and you should get help at once. It's possible that one of the major blood vessels to the eye(s) or to the brain could be blocked.

Treatment: You will probably be admitted to hospital for tests and treatment straightaway. Surgery may sometimes be necessary.

Foggy or blurred vision and/or seeing haloes around lights with aching pain in and above eye

Acute glaucoma, a serious condition in which too much fluid in the eyeball causes pressure to build up, is possible, especially if you are over forty. Seek medical help urgently.

Treatment: You will probably be referred to a hospital specialist right away. Treatment is with eyedrops and other drugs to reduce pressure in the eyeball as quickly as possible. Once the pressure is controlled, surgery may be necessary to prevent the problem recurring.

Blurred vision developing over a period of time

In most cases, gradual blurred vision is caused by eye problems such as short or long-sightedness which can easily be remedied by an optician. After the age of forty, many people notice that their close vision is not as good as it once was. You should have an eye test every two years after this age, as glasses may be needed.

Other disorders such as cataracts or diabetes can cause blurred vision. See your doctor or an optician.

Treatment: An optician will give you a thorough eye test to check your vision and also rule out any underlying eye disease or disorder. Glasses, contact lenses or laser surgery for short-sightedness will be prescribed if necessary. Your doctor may refer you to an optician or to an eye specialist if you have a problem he can't treat.

Sudden blurred vision

Several serious disorders can cause sudden blurred vision. See your doctor at once.

Treatment: Will depend on the cause of the problem.

Flashing lights or floating spots before the eyes

Your doctor may be able to reassure you if symptoms are mild, but you must always consult him. However, a split or tear in the retina, the lining at the back of the eye, is possible, especially if you are very short-sighted or have recently suffered an eye injury. See your doctor at once.

Treatment: Your doctor will probably refer you to a specialist for tests straightaway. Laser surgery is possible if the tear is diagnosed early enough. 'Floaters' also frequently occur before the eyes when there is no underlying abnormality, so if you notice them do not worry unduly, but do have an eye check to be sure.

Flashing lights or floating spots before the eyes followed by headache

Migraine headaches can sometimes cause visual disturbances before they start (see Headache, p. 66).

VOMITING

The most common cause of vomiting is too much rich food or alcohol. However, it's not always a self-inflicted problem.

Anything that gives rise to inflammation or irritation of the stomach or intestine, or disorders that affect the balance mechanism of the inner ear, can cause vomiting. Repeated episodes of vomiting over several days can be caused by persistent inflammation or by ulceration of the stomach lining. Sudden violent vomiting without any prior feelings of sickness or nausea can sometimes be a signal of raised pressure within the skull due to migraine, head injury or inflammation of the brain. Such symptoms should never be ignored, and you should get medical advice immediately.

You should seek urgent medical attention if:

- vomiting is accompanied by headache or severe abdominal pain
- you have vomited on several days in the past week
- you have red or black blood in your vomit
- you have any dark brown matter like coffee grounds (partly digested blood) in your vomit

Vomiting and/or feelings of nausea are common in the early months of pregnancy. If there is any possibility that you could be pregnant, see your doctor. Vomiting can also be caused by certain drugs or medicines taken for other conditions. If you are taking any new medication and suffer from vomiting, consult your doctor.

Abdominal pain with high temperature/ vomiting and/or diarrhoea

Gastroenteritis, an inflammation of the digestive tract due to infection or food poisoning, is likely (see Diarrhoea, p. 51).

Vomiting after eating large amounts of rich, creamy or spicy foods/drinking large amounts of alcohol

An inflammation of the stomach lining, gastritis, can result from eating or drinking too much.

Treatment: Drink plenty of clear fluids in small sips. Eat nothing until the symptoms have subsided. Don't smoke or drink alcohol for at least a day. Don't take aspirin. If the symptoms become worse, or if you are no better within twenty-four hours, see your doctor.

Vomiting with dizziness

A disorder of the inner ear which controls the body's balance mechanisms can cause vomiting. See your doctor.

Treatment: Your doctor may give you medicines which can control the vomiting. He may refer you to a hospital specialist for hearing tests or further investigations.

Severe abdominal pain and vomiting

If you have severe pain that is not relieved by vomiting, a serious condition such as appendicitis or perforated ulcer is possible. Get immediate medical help.

Treatment: Immediate hospital admission is usually needed.

Examination or an operation will be required to discover the cause of the pain and vomiting. An operation may be necessary to remove the appendix or repair an ulcer.

Headache and vomiting

Certain types of migraine can cause vomiting (see Headache, p. 66).

Severe pain in or around one eye and vomiting

Acute glaucoma, excess fluid in the eye which causes pressure to build up, can cause these symptoms (see Vision problems, p. 122).

Recurrent bouts of vomiting and pain in the upper abdomen

An ulcer in the stomach or the duodenum, the pipe that connects it to the intestine, commonly causes such symptoms. See your doctor.

Treatment: If your doctor suspects an ulcer, he may prescribe medicines which will encourage it to heal and reduce the amount of acid in the stomach. He will give you advice about diet and suggest that you eat small, frequent meals and avoid smoking and drinking. He may arrange hospital tests such as an endoscopy or barium X-ray (see Medical diagnostic tests, pp. 304 and 300) to check on the size and site of the ulcer. Sometimes surgery is required to repair an ulcer.

Recurrent bouts of vomiting/loss of appetite/loss of over 10 lbs in last two months

A stomach ulcer or severe gastritis are the most likely cause of these symptoms, but there is also the possibility of stomach cancer. See your doctor at once.

Treatment: Your doctor will arrange for you to have a barium X-ray and/or an endoscopy (see Medical diagnostic tests, pp. 300 and 304). Treatment will depend on the results of these tests.

Recurrent bouts of vomiting and severe pain under ribs on right side of abdomen

Gallstones can cause severe pain when they become stuck in the tube connecting the gallbladder to the digestive tract. See your doctor.

Treatment: Your doctor may arrange for you to have hospital tests such as an ultrasound scan or cholecystography (see Medical diagnostic tests, pp. 308 and 303). If gallstones are diagnosed, you may need an operation to remove the gallbladder. It is sometimes possible to treat gallstones with drugs to dissolve them or with sound waves which shatter them, but this is not suitable in most cases.

Recurrent vomiting with nausea/heartburn/burping

A hiatus hernia, a condition in which part of the stomach protrudes upwards by, or into, the windpipe, can cause these symptoms (see Abdominal pain, p. 19).

Vomiting without nausea/recurrent headaches

Sudden vomiting without the usual feelings of sickness first can occasionally be caused by pressure on the brain. See your doctor at once.

Treatment: Your doctor will probably arrange for tests of the brain such as a CAT scan or radionuclide scan (see Medical diagnostic tests, p. 307). Treatment will depend on the cause of the symptoms.

WEIGHT LOSS

Most people find that their weight dips up and down by a few pounds from time to time, depending on the amount they eat or how much exercise they've taken recently. However, noticeable weight loss (more than 10 lbs (4.5 kg) in two months) that's not the result of dieting or changes in lifestyle should always be referred to your doctor.

Weight loss and loss of appetite with bouts of diarrhoea/bouts of constipation/abdominal pain/blood and/or mucus in faeces

A disorder of the digestive tract such as an inflammation of the intestines or ulceration is likely. There is also the possibility of a tumour. See your doctor at once.

Treatment: Your doctor will refer you to hospital for specialist tests. Samples of blood and faeces may be taken for analysis. A barium X-ray and/or a sigmoidoscopy (see Medical diagnostic tests, pp. 300 and 308) may also be necessary in order to make a diagnosis. Treatment will depend on the diagnosis.

Weight loss accompanied by feeling generally unwell/bouts of raised temperature/frequent sweating at night/persistent cough/blood in phlegm

A chronic lung infection such as tuberculosis (TB) is possible. See your doctor at once.

Treatment: Your doctor will probably need samples of blood and phlegm for analysis. He may also arrange for you to have a chest X-ray. If tuberculosis is diagnosed, the treatment is a long course of antibiotics taken over several months. Most people make a complete recovery and have no further problems.

Weight loss accompanied by increased thirst/ frequent urination/tiredness/genital itching

Diabetes mellitus (sugar diabetes) is a possibility. This is caused when the body fails to produce enough of the hormone insulin, which enables food to be turned into energy. See your doctor at once.

Treatment: Your doctor will take samples of urine and blood for analysis. Mild types of diabetes can be controlled with diet alone. In other cases, daily tablets are required as well, and sometimes injections to provide the insulin that the body is not producing. Insulin can only be given by injection. All diabetic sufferers are instructed carefully on diet and on how to manage their medication.

Loss of weight with normal appetite/excessive sweating/tiredness/weakness or trembling/bulging eyes

An over-active thyroid (thyrotoxicosis) can cause such symptoms.

This is an uncommon condition that mostly affects women. See your doctor.

Treatment: Blood tests and possibly a special scan of the thyroid gland at the base of the neck will be needed to confirm the diagnosis. Treatment is with drugs or, in severe cases, surgery to remove some of the thyroid gland.

WHEEZING

Loud wheezing, especially with breathlessness or painful breathing, can be a sign of several serious conditions and should always be brought to your doctor's attention.

Wheezing accompanied by severe breathing difficulty and feeling as if you are suffocating

A severe attack of asthma is a possibility. If the sufferer becomes bluish around the lips and/or pale and clammy, this is a medical emergency. Call an ambulance or get to hospital at once.

Treatment: Keep the sufferer as calm and comfortable as possible while help arrives. Sitting upright is usually the best position.

Drugs or even a mechanical respirator to help breathing may be given as soon as medical help is on hand.

Wheezing and mild breathing difficulty

A mild attack of asthma is possible. Asthma is a kind of allergic reaction and attacks can be triggered by house dust, animal fur, pollen, and other substances. See your doctor.

Treatment: Your doctor may prescribe drugs to help prevent further attacks and to assist with breathing when they do occur.

Try if possible to discover which things trigger an attack and avoid them in future.

Wheezing and cough with greenish-yellow phlegm on most days

Chronic bronchitis, a persistent inflammation of the lungs and airways, may cause such symptoms. This is especially likely if you are a smoker. See your doctor.

Treatment: Your doctor will probably arrange a chest X-ray for you. Antibiotics may be prescribed to help clear up infection, and possibly other drugs to assist breathing. Smoking is the main cause of chronic bronchitis, and your doctor will strongly advise you to give it up.

Wheezing with raised temperature

Acute bronchitis, an infection of the airways of the lungs, is likely.

Treatment: Stay in a warm environment. Drink plenty of fluids and take aspirin or paracetamol. If you are no better within two days, or if you are worried, see your doctor.

Wheezing and coughing up frothy or pink-stained phlegm

A dangerous build-up of fluid in the lungs is possible. Call medical help at once.

Treatment: Keep calm and sit upright until medical help arrives.

You may be admitted to hospital where you will be given oxygen to help your breathing and drugs to clear fluid from the lungs. When this has been achieved, treatment will depend on the underlying cause of the problem.

WIND

Passing wind either from the mouth or the anus is considered socially embarrassing, but generally causes no more problem than that. Wind is usually the result of the incomplete digestion of foods, which causes excess gases that need to be expelled. Wind may cause an uncomfortable feeling of fullness in the stomach, or make rumbling noises in the intestines. High-fibre foods such as onions, beans and cabbage are common causes of wind, as is beer.

If the problem causes embarrassment, try limiting your intake of these foods.

Wind with an uncomfortable feeling of fullness after meals

Indigestion and wind often go together. They may be caused by eating too fast or by swallowing air while you are eating.

Treatment: Try not to eat meals in a hurry, and allow time to relax after you've eaten. An over-the-counter medicine may help.

If you have severe or frequent attacks of indigestion, see your doctor.

Wind with bouts of lower abdominal pain and/or constipation/diarrhoea

Irritable bowel or diverticular disease can cause these symptoms (see Abdominal pain, p. 22).

Wind with burning pain in centre of chest

A hiatus hernia, a condition in which part of the stomach protrudes upwards, beside or into the gullet, can cause these symptoms (also diagnosed as reflux oesophagitis) when irritant digestive juices splash upwards and inflame the lower end of the gullet (oesophagus) (see Abdominal pain, p. 22).

MEN'S SYMPTOMS

MEN'S SYMPTOMS

Men are fortunate in that they escape the physical complications of pregnancy and childbirth and, because of this, generally need to see their doctor less while they are young. However, there are a number of medical conditions which present specific difficulties for men. Any problems with the urinary system tend to involve men's reproductive organs, and vice versa, because both share a common pathway through the penis – the urethra.

BALDNESS

Hair loss is a natural part of the ageing process. Most men have lost their hair to some extent by the age of sixty, although baldness can begin as early as twenty. Male-pattern baldness is the term used to describe this type of hair loss. Other reasons for hair loss (alopecia) are described below.

Male pattern baldness

Up to 100 hairs are normally shed from the scalp each day, and new hair begins growing in the same hair follicles to replace them. Baldness begins when hair is lost faster than it is replaced. The exact reason why this happens is not known, although it's thought to be linked to an increase in the male hormone androgen, which limits hair growth.

The pattern of male baldness is largely inherited. Sons tend to lose hair at the same age, and in the same areas, as their fathers. A tendency towards early baldness is hereditary. The chances of it increase if there is a history of early baldness on both sides of the family.

Normally, hair loss begins on the temples and crown. Fine, downy hair grows to replace normal hair. Gradually, the affected area widens and baldness increases.

Treatment: Male-pattern baldness is an almost inevitable part of ageing. Until recently, no magic lotions, potions or pills could stop or reverse this type of hair loss. Now, a lotion is available on private prescription which does help in some cases, though it is expensive and has to be used continuously.

There are several ways of concealing baldness. A hair-piece (toupee) is probably the simplest option. Alternatively, hair-weaving, which involves attaching hair-pieces to existing hair, can be successful. Hair transplantation, in which hair from the back or sides of the head is transplanted to the bald patch, is an expensive and often unsatisfactory remedy.

Sudden, patchy hair loss

If the skin of the bald area is scaly and inflamed, a fungal infection such as ringworm may be to blame for patchy hair loss. Often, though, the cause of sudden hair loss when the skin below is perfectly normal is unknown. Some doctors believe this type of hair loss, alopecia areata, which also occurs in women, could be connected with depression and anxiety.

Treatment: Anti-fungal shampoo and/or possibly a course of tablets may be prescribed where a fungal infection is the cause. The hair should return to normal within a few months.

In cases of alopecia areata, there is no specific treatment.

Often the condition disappears of its own accord, and new hair grows within six to nine months. In fact, when it occurs for the first time, four out of five people will recover. Subsequent attacks are less likely to be so short-lived, unfortunately.

DELAYED EJACULATION

Being unable to ejaculate, despite having a normal erection, can be due to physical or emotional problems. Anxiety about sex, worries about pleasing your partner, lack of confidence, fears about maintaining an erection or getting your partner pregnant, can all cause this type of sexual difficulty. In older men, delayed ejaculation, or an occasional inability to ejaculate, is quite normal. Certain drugs or long-term alcohol abuse may inhibit ejaculation. In some cases this problem may be a complication of diabetes.

Treatment: Depends on the reason for the problem. Frank discussion with your partner will help in all cases. Reducing sexual anxiety by relaxing, taking time over love-making, and not feeling under pressure to 'perform', may all help where the problem is emotional in origin. In cases where there is a physical reason for delayed ejaculation, your doctor may be able to remedy the matter.

ERECTION PROBLEMS

Being unable to get an erection, despite being sexually aroused, happens to many men from time to time and is quite normal. It can be due to a variety of causes, both physical and psychological.

Tiredness, stress and anxiety, certain drugs, particularly antidepressants and alcohol abuse, may all cause difficulties with erection. Emotional and psychological problems such as fear of, or anxiety about, having sex, lack of sexual desire, sexual difficulties with a partner, and discord in a relationship, may all cause problems.

Treatment: Depends on the nature of the problem. Emotional and psychological problems can be helped by sexual or relationship counselling. Simple techniques for relaxation and reducing anxiety can usually make a big improvement to a relationship where there are sexual difficulties. Physical problems which cause difficulty with erection can usually be overcome with medical help.

INFERTILITY

The main cause of male infertility is failure to produce enough healthy sperm. Sometimes no sperm at all are produced, and in other cases the sperm are malformed, or don't live long enough to reach the female ova.

Defective sperm may be caused by sexually transmitted diseases which can damage or block the spermatic ducts (see Sexually transmitted diseases, p. 146).

Mumps (see Common childhood infectious illnesses, p. 277) may cause the testes to become painful or swollen, a complication known as orchitis. If a boy has this infection after the age of twelve, it may affect his fertility. Cigarette-smoking, certain drugs and general ill-health or unfitness can reduce fertility. Impotence and disorders affecting ejaculation (see above) may also make it difficult for a man to father a child.

In very rare cases, a chromosomal abnormality or a genetic disease such as cystic fibrosis can be the reason for male infertility.

If your partner has failed to become pregnant after twelve months of having sexual intercourse regularly (twice or three times a week, without using contraception), you should consult your doctor.

Treatment: The doctor will examine you to check on general fitness and state of health and to discover any untreated disorders which could be causing infertility. He may arrange a sperm count test. Treatment for male infertility is limited. If the sperm count is low, artificial insemination may be undertaken to try to achieve pregnancy in his partner.

LOW SEX DRIVE

Not all men have a powerful sex drive. A low level of interest in sex may be perfectly normal in some men, and is no cause for concern provided that it does not create problems in their relationship with a partner. However, an unusual lack of interest in sex can be caused by physical factors such as illness, tiredness or, very occasionally, by a low level of the male sex hormone testosterone. It is much more likely, though, to be due to emotional and psychological factors. Discontent with a relationship, stress, boredom, depression and sexual difficulties can often result in reduced sex drive.

Lack of interest in sex with tiredness/stress

These are very common reasons for loss of interest in sex.

Pressure at work or tiredness after illness can have a detrimental effect on a man's sexual activity.

Self-help measures: Explain to your partner the reasons for your loss of interest in sex. Reassure her that your lack of interest is not due to finding her unattractive. Try to resolve the underlying reasons for your tiredness (see Tiredness, p. 114). When you feel more rested, your normal sex drive should return.

Lack of interest in sex and discontent with the relationship

Disagreements, frequent arguments or general antagonism between partners inevitably result in less interest in sex.

Self-help measures: You must make an effort to tackle these problems by full and frank discussion of your feelings with your partner. Set time aside to talk to each other and fully exchange feelings and ideas. If you can resolve any underlying conflicts, your sexual relationship should improve. Many couples find that they need professional help to sort out long-standing difficulties within a relationship. Seek help from Relate (see Useful addresses, p. 332) if you feel this applies to you.

Specific sexual difficulties

Particular sexual problems can unconsciously make you feel less like sex. Delayed ejaculation (see p. 137) and erection problems (see p. 137) are two common difficulties, but there are many others.

If you feel that a particular problem is affecting your sex life, seek your doctor's advice. He may recommend some professional counselling.

Lack of interest in sex and heavy drinking or taking medicines

Drinking large amounts of alcohol regularly is a common cause of loss of interest in sex. Normal sex drive should return if you cut down or cut out alcohol. If you find this difficult, you should seek your doctor's help. Certain medicines, particularly anti-depressants and anti-anxiety drugs, can cause loss of sex drive. This problem is only temporary and normal interest in sex should return once the course of medication is terminated.

Lack of interest in sex with women

Around 5 per cent of men find that their normal sexual preference is not women, but other men. Many homosexual men are aware of their sexual orientation from early on, but others do not recognize their homosexuality until much later. Society's intolerant attitude towards homosexual men often leads them to repress their sexual feelings, which can result in much unhappiness. If you are experiencing such difficulties, seek your doctor's advice. He will be able to put you in touch with one of the many organizations for gay men that specialize in offering advice and support.

Loss of interest in sex with loss of body hair/ unusually small testes

Very occasionally, loss of interest in sex can be due to lack of the male hormone testosterone. Consult your doctor if low sex drive is accompanied by these additional symptoms.

Treatment: If your doctor suspects this problem, he will refer you for tests to confirm the diagnosis. Hormone treatment is usually successful in correcting the problem.

Loss of interest in sex with ageing

Most men find that their sexual urge diminishes as they grow older.

A need for less frequent sex is common in those over fifty, although this doesn't mean that enjoyment is necessarily reduced.

PAINFUL OR SWOLLEN TESTICLES

Any lumps or swelling in the testicles or of the bag that encloses them, the scrotum, should be reported to your doctor straight-away. Even if it is painless, it could be a symptom of disease, and prompt treatment of any disorder reduces the risk of it developing further or affecting fertility. Men should get into the habit of examining their testes and scrotum once a month for any changes in size, shape or consistency. Cancer of the testes is rare, but can be easily treated if diagnosed early.

Painful testicles

Can be due to a number of causes. Mumps in an adult male can cause an inflammation called orchitis which can cause infertility. Injury to the genitals can cause pain and swelling. Sometimes the testes can twist inside the scrotum (torsion of the testes) and this can be very painful and cause nausea and vomiting.

Treatment: Depends on the cause. There is no specific remedy for orchitis other than painkillers and bed-rest. Damage to the testes as a result of injury may need treatment in hospital, as does torsion of the testes. Both these instances need immediate treatment, possibly including surgery, to avoid the possibility of long-term damage.

One enlarged testicle

This may be due to a cyst, a fluid-filled sac, developing inside the scrotum. Usually these are quite harmless and cause no pain, but you should still be examined by the doctor to rule out the possibility of a tumour – when early treatment is especially important to achieve a cure.

Treatment: A cyst generally requires no treatment unless it becomes so big it is uncomfortable. If the doctor is in any doubt about the swelling, he may refer you for a biopsy (see Medical diagnostic tests, p. 300). A tumour is usually treated by surgical removal.

General painless swelling of the scrotum

A condition called hydrocele is quite common in older men, although it can occur at any age. A clear, thin fluid collects in the scrotum, secreted by the membrane covering the testes and lining the space in which it lies.

Treatment: Your doctor will decide if you need to have the fluid drawn off. This is done under local anaesthetic at the outpatients department of a hospital. If the problem persists, a straightforward operation to stop fluid accumulating there can be performed.

PAINFUL PENIS

A number of different disorders can cause pain in the penis itself, the urinary tract which runs through it, or the skin which covers it. Minor injuries from sport or accidents at work can cause painful bruising or scratches which are not harmful, but any other types of pain or changes in appearance should be seen by a doctor, as should any kind of lump or swelling, even if it's not painful.

Sore blisters, ulcers or sores

These can be caused by sexually transmitted diseases (see p. 146).

Inflammation, redness or swelling on the tip of the penis

This is usually due to an irritation from clothing, or from skin secretions collecting under the foreskin which can set up infection.

Treatment: An antibiotic cream or course of tablets may be prescribed. You'll be instructed to pay special attention to washing carefully under the foreskin.

Painful erection

A painful erection that persists after sexual arousal is known as priapism. It can be caused by a sudden obstruction of the blood vessels that stops blood flowing away from the penis, and can be dangerous.

Treatment: Seek medical help immediately, at a hospital if necessary, if this happens to you. Surgery may be needed to restore normal blood flow, or sometimes drugs can be used. Permanent damage can be done if the condition is not treated promptly.

Pain during or after intercourse

Pain during intercourse can be caused by friction, especially if your partner's vagina is dry.

Soreness after intercourse may be due to friction or possibly to an allergic reaction to a contraceptive cream used by your partner, or to the condom if you use one.

Treatment: Using a lubricating jelly will help prevent soreness from friction during intercourse. If you suspect an allergic reaction, avoid using whatever you think may be causing the problem. If soreness persists, consult your doctor.

Irritating, hard, skin-coloured lumps

These are likely to be anogenital warts caused by a virus that's often, but not always, passed by sexual contact. Don't try to treat the warts yourself, because the skin of the penis is very sensitive.

Treatment: You'll be examined to rule out the possibility of sexually transmitted disease. A cream or paint to apply to the warts will usually be prescribed. You'll be advised to keep the area clean and dry with regular washing, and to avoid sexual contact until the problem has cleared up.

PAINFUL URINATION

If you feel pain or discomfort when passing urine, you should always check with your doctor. It may be a symptom of inflammation or infection.

Painful urination with no other symptoms

A urinary tract infection caused by germs spread from the rectum is the most common cause of this.

Treatment: A sample of urine may be taken for analysis. Treatment usually consists of a course of antibiotics. You'll normally be advised to drink plenty of water.

Painful urination and pain in the lower back

A kidney infection may be the cause of the pain.

Treatment: A sample of urine will probably be taken for analysis. Your doctor may arrange for you to have a special X-ray of the kidneys (intravenous pyelography – see Medical diagnostic tests, p. 306) at a local hospital. A course of antibiotics is normally prescribed for kidney infection in the first instance. Further treatment may be needed depending on the result of tests.

Painful urination with unusual discharge

This can be due to a sexually transmitted infection. See Sexually transmitted diseases, below.

Painful urination and/or pain between the legs, high temperature

Prostatitis, an inflammation of the prostate gland caused by infection, could be the cause.

Treatment: Your doctor will examine you to check if the prostate gland is enlarged. You will be asked for a urine sample.

Antibiotics may be prescribed. If the prostate gland is enlarged and making urination difficult, an operation may be advised.

SEXUALLY TRANSMITTED DISEASES

Sexually transmitted diseases (venereal diseases, VD) are infections passed from one person to another during sexual intercourse, anal and oral sex. Some can damage you, or your partner's, fertility.

The most serious sexually transmitted disease is the human immunodeficiency virus (HIV) that's responsible for the illness AIDS (acquired immune deficiency syndrome). There is no cure for AIDS and it can kill. HIV is on the increase. It is no longer something which affects only homosexual men, but is spreading fast among heterosexual men and women. The more sexual partners you have, the greater is your risk of contracting HIV infection and developing AIDS. The HIV virus lives in the body fluids (blood, semen, vaginal secretions) of infected persons. The only protection against getting or giving the HIV virus is to practise safer sex.

Safer sex is a code of sexual behaviour which aims to reduce the risk of getting or giving the HIV virus. Always wearing a condom is the most important part of safer sex. A condom prevents contact with the body fluids which carry HIV infection.

It is the only protection there is at present against HIV, and using a spermicide in conjunction may give extra protection.

Safer sex also means protecting yourself by restricting the

number of your sexual partners, refusing casual sex, particularly when in parts of the world where AIDS is a particular problem (for example, Central Africa, the West Indies, New York, California), and not indulging in high-risk sexual activities.

High-risk sexual activities are vaginal intercourse without a condom, anal intercourse (even with a condom), any act which draws blood or causes semen or blood to enter the partner's body (oral sex by a woman on a man, for example). There is no risk of contacting HIV from general body contact, stroking, caressing or body kissing.

If you think you may have a sexually transmitted disease, you should get medical help right away, either from your doctor or by attending a sexually transmitted disease clinic at a hospital.

Gonorrhoea

Causes discomfort while passing urine and usually a discharge from the tip of the penis.

Treatment: Once confirmed by taking a sample of discharge for analysis, antibiotics by mouth or injection are prescribed.

Non-specific urethritis (NSU)

A mild tingling at the base of the penis, usually while urinating, and a slight clear discharge are often the only symptoms.

Treatment: A sample of the discharge will be taken for analysis. Treatment is usually a course of antibiotics.

Syphilis

The first sign is a painless sore on the penis, or sometimes around the anus, which is highly infectious. After a couple of weeks this disappears and is replaced by a rash all over the body which does not itch. Sometimes the lymph glands in the armpits swell, and there can also be wart-like lumps in the armpits and around the anus.

Treatment: Syphilis is diagnosed by blood tests and samples taken from sores. The usual treatment is a course of antibiotic injections. Regular blood tests are needed for up to two years afterwards to check that the infection has not re-appeared.

Herpes genitalis

An itchy penis and a crop of small, painful blisters which may spread to the thighs and buttocks are the first signs of herpes. The blisters may burst after a day, leaving small, painful ulcers which crust over. Outbreaks of blisters may recur, the glands in the groin may become enlarged, and the patient may have a high temperature and feel generally unwell.

Treatment: There is no complete cure for herpes. An antiviral drug may make the ulcers less sore and help them to heal.

Pubic lice (crabs)

Itching in the pubic region is the only symptom. The lice, brown and about 1 mm long, may be visible.

Treatment: A lotion or ointment to kill the lice and their eggs will be prescribed.

HIV

The human immunodeficiency virus is responsible for AIDS.

This is a disease which damages the immune system so that the sufferer cannot fight infection. A person becomes HIV-positive after being infected with the HIV virus during sexual or anal intercourse, or from contact with the blood or body fluids of an infected person. Being HIV-positive does not mean that a person will necessarily develop AIDS. Present estimates show that within ten years 50 per cent of HIV-positive people will go on to develop AIDS.

There are not normally any symptoms when a person becomes infected with HIV. The only way of telling if you have been infected is to take a blood test, which shows the presence of HIV antibodies in the blood.

Treatment: There is no cure for the HIV virus. Prevention is the only cure. This means practising safer sex, using a condom, and avoiding coming into contact with the blood or body fluids of HIV-positive people. Intravenous drug-users who share needles, for example, are especially at risk. Advances in treatment have prolonged the life-expectancy of AIDS sufferers by treating the infections they are prone to. Much research is currently under way to improve treatments, but above all to try to develop a vaccine against the HIV virus.

WOMEN'S
SYMPTOMS

WOMEN'S SYMPTOMS

Women are tougher than men – it's a fact. Not only do they live six years longer on average, but they also suffer less coronary heart disease and lung cancer, the two big killers in our society. They have better resistance to disease and to punishing conditions such as cold and exposure. Another plus is that hereditary disorders like haemophilia and colour blindness don't affect women, although of course they can pass them on to their children.

Yet despite the fact that Mother Nature seems to have dealt women a better hand, they are ill more often than men. This is largely due to the one pretty big difference between the sexes – their reproductive systems. Not only is a woman's far more complex than a man's, it also goes through all the changes associated with menstruation, pregnancy and childbirth. So women have an extra set of possible complications to contend with that men don't have to bother about.

BLADDER CONTROL, POOR

This embarrassing problem of urine leaking in the wrong place at the wrong time (urinary incontinence) affects women far more than men. It's especially common at particular stages in a woman's life. The first is after childbirth, when the pelvic-floor muscles have been weakened by the stress of carrying a child. The problem can return at the menopause, when lack of female hormones causes the vagina, bladder and urethra to shrink and lose elasticity. In old age, many women suffer from incontinence who have not done so before, again largely due to muscle weakness. There are several types of incontinence, each due to different causes.

Stress incontinence

Stress incontinence is the escape of a small amount of urine when you laugh, cough, pick up a heavy package, run, or even walk briskly. It's caused by the weakening of the pelvic-floor muscles, which normally hold the exit valve from the bladder, the urethral sphincter, firmly closed. The problem is especially common after childbirth, when the pelvic-floor muscles have been over-stretched.

A prolapsed womb or vagina, where the womb has dropped down out of position or the vaginal walls have bulged due to pressure from other organs, may also cause stress incontinence. Again, the culprit is weakened pelvic-floor muscles. With a pro-lapse, however, there are usually other symptoms, such as a dragging-down feeling in the pelvis and/or backache.

Treatment: Your doctor will first take a urine specimen to rule out infection or diabetes. Infection may be treated with anti-biotics. Diabetes needs more thorough investigation.

Pelvic-floor exercises to tone and strengthen the pelvic muscles can be a great help. They must be done correctly, regularly, and for at least three months before results start to show. Your doctor may suggest that you diet if you are overweight, because this can add to the problems of stress incontinence. You may be referred to a specially trained continence advisor at a local hospital for further help and advice.

Surgery to strengthen, or take a tuck in, the pelvic-floor muscles is sometimes possible if exercises don't bring results, although it's not advisable until after a woman's family is complete.

In cases of prolapse, a specially designed vaginal pessary, in addition to the pelvic-floor exercises, can help until surgery to repair the prolapse is recommended.

Urge incontinence/unstable bladder/ irritable bladder

A condition in which the bladder becomes over-sensitive, and even small amounts of urine cause an urgent need to urinate. The reason for the problem isn't always clear. It can be due to the menopause, but stress, emotional problems, and poor bladder training may also spark it off. Any damage to the nervous system – a stroke, spinal injury or multiple sclerosis – can disrupt the reflex mechanisms that govern bladder control. Diabetes and bladder infections can also cause abnormally frequent urination.

Treatment: Re-training the bladder to ignore the urge to urinate can help. In some cases, drugs to relax the bladder muscles and calm the nerves that control contractions may be prescribed.

Your doctor may refer you for tests. These may include X-rays to rule out kidney stones, an ultrasound scan for information about the bladder, cystoscopy (see Medical diagnostic tests, p. 303) or cystometry – a series of bladder-function tests that measure the volume and pressure of the bladder.

Sudden loss of bladder control

This may be due to damage to the spinal cord or nervous system, especially if you've recently suffered a back injury or experienced weakness in your legs. Seek medical help at once.

Treatment: Depends on the diagnosis.

Inability to pass urine

If you find you're unable to pass urine even though you feel the urge, you should seek medical help urgently. You may have an obstruction which could be serious.

Treatment: Depends on the diagnosis.

BREAST PROBLEMS

Pain, tenderness and the development of lumps are the commonest breast complaints. These problems, including harmless lumps, are generally minor and easily treated. However, breast lumps or humps should always be taken seriously, because breast cancer is one of the most common cancers in women, responsible for 15,000 deaths in the UK each year. This is why it's so important to examine your breasts every month to check for any changes, particularly if you're over forty. And if you're aged between fifty and sixty-four the NHS mammogram X-ray programme will offer you screening every three years.

Pain and tenderness

Tingling and discomfort, a feeling of fullness, heaviness or tenderness, are common and quite normal before periods, around puberty, in early pregnancy and, for some women, during the first few months of taking the contraceptive pill. This is thought to be because increased levels of the female hormones oestrogen or progesterone cause the cells of the breast to retain more fluid than usual. Some women also suffer breast pain in the years before the menopause. The most common breast lumps, fibroadenosis, are fluid-filled cysts which make the breasts feel tender and lumpy in the week or two before a period (see below).

Breast cancer rarely causes pain.

Treatment: No treatment is normally necessary. A good supporting bra can make the breasts feel more comfortable. Hormone treatments can be prescribed for severe pre-menstrual problems, and they can also help with benign breast lumps. Your doctor will examine you and refer you for a mammogram if there is any cause for concern. Cysts are treated by drawing off the fluid through a syringe.

Lumps

A single, firm, painless lump, or a group of them that feel rubbery and can be moved about in the breast, can be a cyst, caused by a secretory gland's blocked duct or fibroadenomas. This is a group of lumps often caused by the milk glands thickening up. Many women have slightly lumpy breasts just before a period.

They may feel as if a lot of little orange-pips are just under the skin.

All these conditions are benign breast diseases and are not harmful. However, a painless lump in the breast or armpit is also the most common sign of breast cancer and should never be ignored. Only one in ten breast lumps are due to cancer, but all lumps need examining immediately by your doctor. If you are breastfeeding and develop a single very painful lump and inflammation, you could have a breast abscess or mastitis.

Treatment: Your doctor will examine you and arrange a special-ist test, a mammogram, biopsy (see Medical diagnostic tests, pp. 307 and 300) or aspiration (withdrawal of fluid) if there's any cause for concern. Painful fibroadenomas are usually treated with hormones or may be removed by surgery if they cause prob-lems. Cysts are treated by drawing off the fluid with a syringe, usually under local anaesthetic. Antibiotics may be prescribed if there is any infection.

Breast cancer may be treated by surgery, chemotherapy and/or radiotherapy. Breast abscesses are treated with antibiotics.

Mastitis usually only occurs at times when the breasts are tense with milk. A firm supporting bra, continuing to feed the baby and expressing excess milk will be recommended.

Discharge from the nipple

Any sort of unexpected fluid coming from the nipple should never be ignored. A clear or blood-stained discharge could poss-ibly be due to a cyst. But it could also be a symptom of a more serious tumour. Your must check with your doctor.

Treatment: Your doctor will examine you and arrange the specialist tests described above if there's any cause for concern. Treatment will depend on the cause of the discharge.

Drawn in nipple/puckered skin/itchy nipple

Any of these symptoms need investigation by your doctor. There may be a perfectly simple explanation, but they could also be caused by a tumour.

Treatment: Depends on what's causing the problem.

Large breasts/small breasts

There's a great variation in the size of breasts, and nearly all sizes are perfectly normal. It is very common to have one breast larger than the other. Small breasts work just as well as large ones when it comes to feeding a baby, although breasts enlarge considerably during pregnancy. A good, well-fitting support bra is essential for large breasts, and can work wonders for small ones too.

Treatment: Hormone treatment may help some women whose breasts have failed to develop during puberty. Plastic surgery can be successful for both very large and very small breasts.

CONTRACEPTION

It is still the woman who takes responsibility for contraception in most relationships. This may be because more choices of contraception are open to her, or because an unwanted pregnancy will affect her far more than her partner. Contraception, the control of fertility to prevent pregnancy, works in one of three ways: by stopping the production of an egg (ovum) in the woman (the combined contraceptive pill, hormone injections); by preventing sperm from meeting an ovum (the diaphragm (cap), the sponge,

the condom, the progestogen-only pill, female sterilization, vasec-
tomy, 'natural' family planning methods); or by preventing a
fertilized egg from implanting in the uterus (IUDs, the 'morning
after' pill).

Most methods of contraception have advantages and disadvantages; some carry slight risks, and not all are suitable for all
women. Several factors have to be weighed up when choosing a
method of contraception. Most women find that they will change
methods several times during their fertile years, depending on
which is most convenient and suitable for their needs at a given
time.

The contraceptive pill

There are two types of contraceptive pill – the combined pill and
the progestogen-only pill.

The combined pill contains two hormones, oestrogen and progestogen. Taken regularly, it mainly stops ovulation (the release
of a woman's egg each month). The pill is virtually 100 per cent
effective when taken correctly (far fewer than one pregnancy per
100 women using this method for one year). Other potential
advantages are regular menstrual bleeding and reduced period
pain and pre-menstrual tension. Its main disadvantages are side-
effects for some women – headaches, depression, increased blood
pressure and weight gain. Some research studies have suggested
that long-term use of the combined pill may cause an increased
risk of cervical and breast cancers, while others have shown that
it protects against cancers of the womb and ovaries.

The progestogen-only pill contains only the hormone progestogen. It causes thickening of the mucus in the cervix at the
entrance to the womb, and so prevents sperm reaching the ovum.

It can be almost as effective as the combined pill if taken correctly, at exactly the same time every day (one pregnancy per
100 women a year). Side-effects and possible health risks seem
to be fewer than with the combined pill.

Hormone injections

These work in a similar way to the progestogen-only pill and also prevent ovulation. The hormone progestogen is injected into a muscle and is slowly released over eight or twelve weeks.

This method is very effective (fewer than one pregnancy per 100 women a year), but only considered suitable for women who can't use other methods of contraception. It causes periods to become irregular, and fertility may take up to one year to return after its use.

Intra-uterine device (IUD or coil)

This small device, usually made of plastic and copper, is inserted into the womb by a doctor. It works in several ways, by preventing a fertilized egg settling in the womb or by preventing an egg and sperm meeting. It is very effective (one to three pregnancies per 100 women per year), especially if used with a spermicide. Side-effects may include heavier periods and an increased risk of pelvic infection. The IUD needs to be replaced about every five years. It is not usually recommended for young women who have never been pregnant.

The diaphragm (cap)

This is a soft rubber device which is inserted high into the vagina before intercourse to cover the cervix. It prevents sperm from meeting the ovum. It must be used with spermicide and left in place for six hours after intercourse. It can be very reliable if used conscientiously (two pregnancies per 100 women per year) and has the advantage of no side-effects. However, it is not as convenient as other methods since it must be inserted before intercourse and may interfere with love-making.

The female condom

A fine polyurethane sheath, closed at one end to cover the cervix, that's inserted into the vagina. The open end has a ring that stays outside the vagina to stop the condom slipping inside during intercourse.

Like the male condom, it prevents sperm reaching the ovum and has the advantage of protecting against sexually transmitted disease. Studies show the female condom is between 88–98 per cent effective at preventing pregnancy.

The condom (sheath)

A thin rubber tube worn over the erect penis that prevents sperm entering the woman. Its advantages are that it's safe and easy to use, and also offers protection to both partners against sexually transmitted diseases, including HIV.

It is as effective as the diaphragm or IUD (two pregnancies per 100 women per year) if used carefully. The disadvantages are that the condom can slip off during love-making, and some couples find it an inconvenience to use.

The sponge

A soft, circular foam sponge containing spermicide that is inserted into the vagina up to twenty-four hours before love-making to cover the cervix. It must be left in place for six hours after intercourse and is effective for twenty-four hours. The sponge is easy to use and has no side-effects, but it is one of the least reliable contraceptive methods (nine pregnancies per 100 women per year).

Female sterilization

A permanent method of contraception for women who are certain that they've completed their family. The Fallopian tubes are closed so that an egg cannot travel down them to meet sperm. The operation usually entails a day in hospital.

This is the most reliable contraceptive method of them all. Very, very rarely (one pregnancy per 1,000 sterilizations) the Fallopian tubes re-join and fertility returns.

Natural methods

These aim to predict the time that a woman ovulates so that intercourse can be avoided during her fertile days. The two main methods are the sympto-thermal method, which relies largely on a daily temperature check, and the Billings method, which involves noting changes in cervical mucus. Both methods require careful record-keeping and a high degree of commitment from both partners.

GENITAL IRRITATION

Itching or soreness of the vagina or around the vulva (the external genital area) is known medically as pruritus vulvae. If the itching isn't accompanied by an abnormal or unpleasant vaginal discharge (see Vaginal discharge, p. 184, and Sexually transmitted diseases, p. 179) the most likely cause is a skin irritation or a change in hormone levels.

Sore, irritated skin

The skin around the genital area is delicate and needs to be treated gently. It is lubricated by secretions from the vaginal glands which keep it moist and soft. Perfumes and chemicals in harsh soaps, deodorants, bath salts and cleansers may disturb the skin's natural chemical balance and cause drying and irritation.

Treatment: The genital area should be washed daily as part of normal hygiene, but use plain warm water only. Vaginal douches and deodorants are unnecessary and should be avoided. Also steer clear of talcum powders, bath salts and perfumed soaps. Try to avoid the temptation to scratch the area; it will make matters worse. Cotton underwear is preferable to man-made fibres; it allows the skin to breathe. Also avoid tights and tight trousers which may rub and make the skin hot. If the irritation persists for more than two weeks, see your doctor.

Sore, irritated or tender skin

When the level of female hormones decreases around the time of the menopause, less lubricating mucus may be secreted. The result is that the vagina can become sore, dry and tender. There may be soreness and discomfort particularly during intercourse.

Treatment: Follow the general advice given above and seek your doctor's advice. He may prescribe a hormone cream to apply to the vagina and vulva, or suggest that you consider hormone replacement therapy. A lubricating jelly used before sexual intercourse can help avoid soreness.

INFERTILITY

Infertility affects as many as one in six couples, and becomes more common with age. It can be due to a problem with either the male or the female partner, although far more is known about female infertility, and medical investigations tend to concentrate on the woman. The most common reasons for female infertility are failure to produce eggs (ovulate) and blocked Fallopian tubes.

Fibroids, pelvic infection, and endometriosis (see Periods, p. 173) can also prevent or delay conception. Infertility also occurs when a woman's cervical mucus is hostile to her partner's sperm and produces antibodies that kill or immobilize it. The major known cause of male infertility is failure to produce enough healthy sperm.

Discovering the cause of infertility often requires intensive investigation, usually in a specialist hospital clinic.

If you have been having regular intercourse for over a year without contraception and haven't become pregnant, you should consult your doctor. Some doctors suggest that women over thirty should take advice after six months. A woman's fertility begins to decline after this age, and there is less time for investigation and treatment should it be needed.

There are several steps that can be taken to increase the chances of conception. When both partners are in good health, fertility is higher. A good diet, plenty of rest and exercise, and restricting smoking and drinking are good ways to improve general health.

Have intercourse about three times a week. This way you will be sure that you don't miss your most fertile days, just before and after an egg is produced. Ovulation testing-kits are available at the chemist's. These predict when a woman is about to ovulate by testing urine. Using them, a woman can maximize her chances of conceiving by timing intercourse for her most fertile period.

After intercourse, remain lying down for fifteen minutes to allow the maximum number of sperm to enter the womb.

Men should not wear tight underpants which may increase the temperature inside the scrotum and damage sperm.

Blocked Fallopian tubes

The Fallopian tubes lead from the ovaries to the womb on either side. Their job is to guide an egg from the ovary to the womb. There are several ways in which they can become damaged or diseased, making the passage of an egg difficult or impossible. Pelvic inflammatory disease (PID), that is any chronic inflammation of the pelvic organs, can cause the Fallopian tubes to become scarred and blocked or narrowed.

Sexually transmitted diseases such as gonorrhoea and chlamydia (see pp. 181–2) are one of the commonest causes of PID. It can also occasionally flare up after a miscarriage, abortion or childbirth.

An ectopic pregnancy, where a fertilized egg implants itself in the Fallopian tube, can also cause damage and prevent later conception.

Treatment: A specialist investigation called a laparoscopy (see Medical diagnostic tests, p. 306) will probably be carried out under general anaesthetic to confirm the diagnosis. The procedure is also sometimes used to clear minor blockages of the Fallopian tubes. If this fails, surgery to clear blocked tubes is sometimes successful.

Failure to ovulate

Anovulation (failure to ovulate) is the most common cause of female infertility. Absent periods (see Periods, p. 170) are a sign that you are not producing an egg each month. However, some women do have periods without producing an egg.

Severe stress, strenuous exercise, anorexia nervosa (even overdieting), a hormone imbalance, or a disorder of the ovary such as a tumour or cyst may all prevent ovulation.

Treatment: Investigations will be carried out to discover why an egg is not being produced each month. These may include a laparoscopy, ultrasound scan (see Medical diagnostic tests, pp. 306 and 308), blood and urine analysis, and keeping a monthly temperature chart. Treatment depends on the reason for the failure to ovulate. Surgery may be suggested for ovarian cysts, or hormone treatment to stimulate the ovaries to produce an egg if this is appropriate.

In vitro fertilization (IVF)

When normal fertility treatments fail or are inappropriate, *in vitro* fertilization may offer the chance of a child to some couples. The procedure involves giving drugs to stimulate the woman's ovaries into producing a number of eggs, which are then collected using a hollow needle inserted into her abdomen. The eggs are then mixed with sperm in a test-tube, and the fertilized embryos inserted into the woman's womb. In another method, GIFT (gamete intra-Fallopian transfer), the ova are mixed with sperm and injected directly into the Fallopian tube rather than fertilized outside the woman's body.

Both methods are physically and emotionally demanding for the couple involved and have a high failure rate. Success rates vary, but estimates suggest that although 25 per cent of women become pregnant after IVF, only 10 per cent deliver a live baby. Multiple births, with all the risks that they involve, are also quite common with IVF.

Demand for the treatment far outstrips the available NHS facilities. There are long waiting-lists. Many privately-run centres offer the costly procedure, some excellent and some not so good.

It's important to be properly examined before embarking on IVF. This is because some causes of infertility can be remedied without expensive IVF treatment. It is alleged that some un-scrupulous private clinics will advise IVF even when it is completely unsuitable.

In vitro fertilization is a controversial method of conceiving a child, and some people have moral and ethical objections to it.

PAINFUL INTERCOURSE

Pain or discomfort in or around the vagina or deep within the pelvis during intercourse is known medically as dyspareunia. It can happen to women of any age and may be due to a variety of physical or emotional problems.

Soreness of the vagina

Soreness or bruising of the vagina is quite common after a first or a new sexual relationship, or because of very enthusiastic sex.

It is also quite normal after childbirth, especially if there have been stitches for an episiotomy repair. The lining of the vagina and/or stitches may take at least six weeks to heal. In older women, the hormonal changes associated with the menopause can cause the lining of the vagina to become thinner and less well lubricated. This can make intercourse uncomfortable or sometimes even painful.

Treatment: Soreness as the result of unaccustomed or very frequent sex is no cause for concern. Abstaining from sex for a day or so will help.

After childbirth a medical check at six weeks should make sure that all stitches and internal tears are fully healed. If discomfort persists for longer, go back to your doctor for help. A lubricating jelly can help ease the soreness in the early months after childbirth. At the menopause, lubricating jelly may also help. Alternatively, your doctor may consider prescribing hormone replacement therapy.

Dry, tight vagina

Lack of arousal during love-making prevents lubrication of the vagina and relaxation of the surrounding muscles and tissues. Penetration is then painful or even impossible. Usually, the reason for this is an emotional or psychological one, although menopausal changes can cause dryness too (see above). Tiredness, stress or tension, or anxiety caused by shame or fear, anger or resentment towards one's partner, may be to blame.

Treatment: Self-help measures aimed at relaxation and reducing anxiety before intercourse is attempted can often help. These include a gentle, unhurried approach, enough time and privacy to unwind, even warm baths and relaxing massage. If such measures fail, your doctor may check to rule out any physical cause for the problem. He may put you in touch with an organization or a doctor offering sexual counselling or marriage guidance. These can be very successful in overcoming such difficulties when both partners are committed to it.

Vaginal spasm

Some women suffer an involuntary spasm of the pelvic-floor
muscles when intercourse is attempted. This almost completely
closes the vaginal opening, making penetration impossible. This
spasm is called vaginismus. A high level of sexual anxiety due to
guilt, fear, or sometimes a shocking experience such as rape, is
often the underlying reason for this uncommon problem.

Treatment: Once your doctor has ruled out a physical cause
being responsible for this disorder, he will probably suggest that
you seek marriage guidance or sex therapy, and will put you in
touch with a suitable organization or doctor.

Pain on penetration

Pain deep in the pelvis during sexual intercourse can be due to
a number of pelvic problems.

Endometriosis (p. 173), fibroids (p. 173), ovarian cysts (p. 165),
pelvic inflammatory disease (p. 174), cystitis (p. 169), cervical
infections or tumours (p. 183), or enlarged pelvic veins can all
be responsible for pelvic pain.

Treatment: Depends on the underlying cause of the pain.

Antibiotics may be prescribed for infection. Drugs and/or surgery are possible courses of action for the other disorders.

PAINFUL OR FREQUENT URINATION

Most of us need to use the lavatory between twice and six times
a day. If you find that you are needing to go more often, or that
passing urine is painful, you may need to seek your doctor's help.

Passing large amounts of pale urine

If you have recently become unusually thirsty, and have also felt very tired, suffered weight loss, and possibly some genital irritation, you should see your doctor. Diabetes is a possibility. This disorder is caused when the body fails to produce enough of the hormone insulin, needed to make energy from the sugars and carbohydrate foods we eat.

Treatment: Your doctor will want to take blood and urine tests if he suspects that diabetes is a possibility. If the diagnosis is confirmed, you may be able to control the illness with diet, or may need to take tablets or injections depending on its severity. You will probably be referred to a diabetic clinic at a hospital for full dietary and treatment advice if you need to take tablets or injections of insulin.

Frequent urge to urinate but passing only small amounts

Increased frequency of urination is one of the earliest symptoms of pregnancy. It usually passes after the first three months, but may return towards the end of the pregnancy as the baby grows larger and presses on the bladder. An unstable bladder (see Bladder control, poor, p. 153) gives a strong urge to urinate even when only small amounts of urine are present.

Treatment: No treatment is necessary in the case of pregnancy.

For unstable bladder, tests and treatment may be offered (see p. 155).

Frequent, painful urination

Either an inflammation of the bladder (cystitis) or an inflammation of the urethra (urethritis) is the most likely cause. Both can be, but are not always, due to an infection. The urine may also sometimes be cloudy, blood-stained or strong-smelling. This is not usually any cause for concern.

Treatment: Your doctor may ask for a specimen of urine to check for infection. He may prescribe antibiotics or a medicine to make your urine less acid. He will probably suggest that you drink plenty of fluids but avoid very sweet drinks. Soluble aspirin or paracetamol and a hot-water bottle can help relieve any pain or discomfort you may have in the lower abdomen.

Painful urination with pain in the small of the back just above the waist

You should see your doctor straightaway, especially if you have a temperature too, because these symptoms could mean that you have an infection of the kidneys which needs immediate treatment.

Treatment: Your doctor will ask for a urine sample for analysis.

He will probably prescribe antibiotics and give you the advice outlined above for cystitis. If you frequently suffer from this type of infection, he may refer you to hospital for further tests such as blood analysis or an intravenous pyelography (see Medical diagnostic tests, p. 306) to discover if there is any underlying cause.

PERIODS

Absent

The medical term for absent periods is amenorrhoea. In young women whose periods have never started at all, it is known as primary amenorrhoea. In women who usually have normal periods and then miss several consecutively, it is known as secondary amenorrhoea. Missing periods are not normally any cause for concern. Pregnancy is the most common reason in normally healthy and sexually active women.

No periods ever

Menstruation normally starts sometime between the ages of ten and fifteen. It can start later for some girls, though, especially in those of below-average height or weight. If a girl has not begun periods by the age of sixteen, primary amenorrhoea is diagnosed.

The main reason for primary amenorrhoea is delayed puberty, though often the other developments will have occurred normally – breast development for example.

There's not normally any serious reason for the menstrual delay. Occasionally it can be due to a disorder of the endocrine system – the glands and organs responsible for producing the hormones which regulate body functions. An under-active thyroid gland can sometimes be the cause of delayed puberty.

When the eating disorders anorexia nervosa and bulimia, which affect as many as one in 100 young women, cause weight loss to below that which is normal for the person's age and height, the hormone balance can, and usually will, be disrupted. This can cause periods to stop, or never to start at all. Even slightly over-dieting can have this effect too.

Treatment: The doctor will give a complete physical examination to check that development is normal, and may arrange for blood tests to measure hormone levels. Usually no treatment is necessary – puberty, though delayed, will soon arrive. However, if the problem is due to a hormone disorder, further investigations and possible hormone treatment are usually carried out by a specialist.

If anorexia nervosa or bulimia is the cause, treatment is needed urgently, because of the long-term general threat to health.

Missed periods

If you have missed one or more periods, and you are sure that you are not pregnant, there may be several other simple explanations. Stress, illness, emotional upheaval, or strenuous physical activity such as athletic training, can all disrupt the menstrual cycle.

Periods are usually irregular after childbirth, and when a woman is breastfeeding regularly they usually stop altogether. Beware, however – this does not mean that you can't become pregnant, since an ovum may still be produced during this time.

In the years leading up to the menopause, irregular and missed periods are also normal.

If you have recently stopped taking the contraceptive pill, it may take some time to re-establish a regular cycle again. See your doctor if your periods haven't returned after two months.

The eating disorders anorexia nervosa and bulimia – should this latter condition cause weight loss – can also cause periods to stop.

Missing periods are not in themselves a cause for concern, except in the case of eating disorders, but if they are due to feeling generally unwell, run-down or anxious, you should seek your doctor's advice.

Treatment: None is normally necessary, except in the case of eating disorders, which require urgent specialist help because of the long-term threat to health. Your doctor may give you a general health check and advise on taking better care of yourself if you are run-down.

Heavy

Every woman's menstrual cycle is different – the amount of blood lost and the time it lasts varies. However, on average, bleeding lasts for five days, with the heaviest flow occurring in the first three days. If you begin to lose more blood than you usually do, if bleeding lasts longer than normal, or if you need to change your sanitary protection much more often than usual, you should see your doctor. The medical term for heavy periods is menorrhagia.

Regularly heavy periods
If your periods have always been heavy, you may have a thicker womb lining (endometrium) than most women.

This is not in itself a cause for concern, but you should see your doctor if the problem is troublesome. Alternatively, a hormone imbalance may be responsible, although this is quite rare and is more likely to cause occasional heavy periods.

Treatment: Your doctor may take a blood sample to check that frequent heavy blood-loss is not causing anaemia. Iron tablets and dietary advice will be given if it is. He may suggest a D & C (dilation and curettage) operation.

This is a minor operation performed under general anaesthetic in hospital to investigate the cause of heavy periods, among other things. The cervix is dilated and the womb lining is scraped away. In some cases it may cure the problem of heavy periods.

Another possible course of action is hormone treatment. Your doctor may suggest that you try the contraceptive pill even though you may not need this for contraceptive purposes, as it will reduce the blood loss.

One heavy period

If you have an unusually heavy period that's also late, and especially if it's painful too, it's possible that you may have suffered an early miscarriage, although normal periods, from time to time, may be very heavy.

Treatment: If you think you may have had a miscarriage, consult your doctor. No special action may be necessary, but he will want to check that all is well.

Heavy, painful periods

If your periods are heavy, last longer than usual, contain clots of blood, and especially if they're also painful, fibroids could be to blame. These are harmless fibrous growths in the lining of the womb, and can be as small as a pea or as large as a grapefruit. They are very common in women over thirty-five; by the age of forty-five, one in five women has fibroids.

Small fibroids often cause no trouble, and many women are not even aware of them, but larger ones may need treatment.

Endometriosis, where the tissue of the lining of the womb forms outside the womb, causing pain and increased bleeding, is also a possibility.

Treatment: Small fibroids that don't cause any trouble can be safely left alone. If there are troublesome symptoms, drug treatment may be prescribed to reduce bleeding.

Large, troublesome fibroids which don't respond to drug treatment are usually removed by surgery. A myomectomy, which removes only the fibroids, may be offered to younger women who want children. A hysterectomy is more likely to be offered to older women and those who have completed their family. There is also a newer procedure, TCRE (transcervical resection of the endometrium), which permanently removes the womb lining.

Fibroids tend to shrink naturally after the menopause, when the action of the female hormone oestrogen, which makes them grow faster, has stopped. Older women are therefore sometimes advised to 'wait and see' if the problem solves itself.

Endometriosis is usually treated by long-term hormone therapy.

Irregular

A typical monthly cycle lasts twenty-eight days, but normal menstrual cycles may vary from twenty-four to thirty-one days between periods. If the time between periods varies widely each month, then your periods are irregular.

For the first few years after a young woman starts her periods, and for the few years leading up to the menopause, irregular periods are very common (see Absent periods, p. 170).

An upset in the menstrual pattern may be caused by many different things: stress, travel, changing your method of contraception, a hormone imbalance, or sometimes an underlying disorder such as fibroids (p. 173), ovarian cysts (p. 165), endometriosis (p. 173), or pelvic inflammatory disease (see below).

Irregular periods should not be confused with spotting or vaginal bleeding between periods (p. 183). This can be a symptom of a more serious disorder of the womb or cervix, and should not be ignored.

Treatment: May not be necessary if there is no underlying disorder. Otherwise, treatment will depend on the cause of the problem.

Irregular painful periods with backache, pain during intercourse, vaginal discharge

These are the main symptoms of pelvic inflammatory disease and should never be ignored. PID is an infection of the female reproductive organs and can affect the Fallopian tubes, ovaries or uterus. It can be difficult to get rid of once it gets a hold, and it tends to recur. It can in severe cases cause scarring of the Fallopian tubes, leading to infertility. The infection can be caused by sexually transmitted diseases such as chlamydia (p. 182) or gonorrhoea (p. 181). It can also occur after miscarriage, abortion or childbirth. IUD-users and sexually active young women have a higher rate of PID than others.

Treatment: A doctor will examine you and take a smear to identify the type of infection. Antibiotics will be prescribed to clear it up. In severe cases, a laparoscopy (see Medical diagnostic tests, p. 306) may be performed to check the diagnosis and the extent of the infection.

In very severe cases of PID that don't respond to other treatments, a hysterectomy may be suggested.

Painful

Painful periods (primary dysmenorrhoea) affect about one third of all women between the ages of fifteen and twenty-five. The pain is due to a muscle spasm of the womb, almost like a mini-labour. It's thought to be the result of the body producing too much of the hormone prostaglandin, or because the sufferer is especially sensitive to this hormone. It's not an old wives' tale that painful periods usually disappear after a woman has her first baby.

In women over thirty, painful periods (secondary dysmenorrhoea) are more likely to be due to an underlying disorder of the womb, or to an infection.

Stomach cramps, dull ache in the abdomen or back
The pain usually starts before the period or on the first day, and gets easier as the period goes on. Some women experience vomiting, headache and diarrhoea also. Pain may be so bad that bed-rest is needed.

Treatment: Hot-water bottles, hot baths and aspirin are traditional remedies for period pain, and can bring considerable relief. Ibuprofen (Nurofen) is a painkiller with an anti-prostaglandin effect that can be particularly helpful. A doctor can prescribe stronger anti-prostaglandin drugs and anti-spasmodic medicines. The contraceptive pill is often suggested for painful periods, and can eliminate the symptoms for many women.

Painful periods with heavy bleeding
Fibroids (p. 173), endometriosis (p. 173), or ovarian cysts (p. 165) can all be responsible for increased pain and bleeding in older women.

Treatment: Your doctor may perform an internal examination or send you for an ultrasound scan (see Medical diagnostic tests, p. 308) in hospital to help diagnose the problem.

Treatment will depend on the cause of the symptoms.

Painful periods with abnormal vaginal discharge and low back pain
Pelvic inflammatory disease is a possibility (p. 174). See your doctor as soon as possible.

SEX, LOSS OF INTEREST IN

Everyone differs in the amount of sex that they find normal and satisfying. Some women like to have sex every day, others once a week, once a month or less often; all are normal patterns.

However, suddenly becoming less interested in sex, or not wanting it at all, may be a sign of a number of physical or emotional problems that often need help, not least because of the bad effect that loss of interest in sex can have on a relationship.

Illness, tiredness, stress

These can all lead to a lack of interest in sex which is usually temporary. Virus illnesses such as influenza and glandular fever especially can have this effect.

Treatment: None is usually necessary. Once recovery is complete, or the stressful or hard-working episode is over, interest in sex should return quite naturally. However, see your doctor if loss of interest or other symptoms persist.

Childbirth

The birth of a baby is well known to ruin the sex life of its parents, at least temporarily. After childbirth, a woman is usually physically and emotionally drained for some weeks or even months. Stitches may be sore, and the exhaustion involved in caring for a small baby, with many broken nights, takes its toll.

Treatment: Is not normally necessary provided that there is no physical cause for the loss of interest. Usually, a check six weeks after the birth will confirm that all is healing normally. A lubricating jelly can help if painful intercourse is the reason for avoiding it. Tiredness may persist for many months. If intercourse is infrequent or non-existent during this time, it's important that partners show their care and affection for each other in other ways, by cuddling, holding, or mutual masturbation.

The important point is that neither partner should suffer feelings of rejection, or resentment towards the new baby.

Hormonal disorders

Changes in your menstrual pattern which cause irregular (p. 174) or missed periods (p. 171) may also cause a lack of interest in sex. An under-active thyroid may also cause lack of energy and low sex drive.

Treatment: If your doctor suspects a hormone imbalance, he may send blood samples for analysis. Treatment will depend on the cause of the problem.

Depression

Loss of interest in sex is a classic symptom of depression. Depression may be brought on by a stressful event such as divorce, bereavement, or job loss. It may also cause trouble sleeping, early waking, or feelings of guilt, inadequacy and hopelessness (see Depression, p. 47).

Pre-menstrual tension may cause some women to feel especially low in the days before their period.

Treatment: Will depend on the reasons for, and nature of, the depression. Anti-depressant drugs, counselling and psychotherapy are the most usual treatments. In cases of severe depression, it may be necessary to spend some time in hospital for extensive treatment. Pre-menstrual tension may sometimes be treated with hormone therapy. Some women find a diet rich in the vitamin B6, found in liver, chicken, whole grains, wheatgerm and bananas helpful.

Fear of getting pregnant

Concern about an unwanted pregnancy can put women off sex. Good, reliable contraceptive precautions can overcome this problem (see Contraception, p. 158).

Treatment: See your doctor or attend a family planning clinic to discuss the most suitable type of contraception for your needs.

Sexual difficulties

Specific sexual difficulties, such as failure to achieve orgasm in the woman, premature ejaculation or impotence in the man, may cause loss of interest in sex.

Treatment: You will need to discuss the problem fully and frankly with your doctor before he can help.

He may offer advice, arrange for you to see a counsellor, or refer you to an organization offering sexual counselling, such as

RELATE (see Useful Addresses, p. 332), or to a specialist doctor suggested by the Family Planning Clinic. Sexual counselling and therapy take many forms depending on the nature of the problem. Usually, talking frankly about feelings and problems is a large part of the programme. There may also be physical exercises for partners to carry out to overcome specific problems. Sex therapy and counselling can be very successful in overcoming problems when both partners are committed to them and to their relationship.

Relationship problems

Resentment, antagonism, hostility and dislike between partners reduce their mutual physical attraction and desire. Sex is often the first casualty in a failing relationship.

Treatment: The best remedy is to talk out problems and to try to come to agreement about a course of action to rectify matters. In many relationships in trouble, though, lack of communication between partners is one of the major difficulties. Such couples can benefit enormously from the help of trained counsellors to help them express their feelings and get to the root of difficulties.

Marriage guidance counsellors can be contacted through RELATE (see Useful addresses, p. 332). Their help can be vital in saving failing marriages. The address of a local doctor trained in psychosexual medicine can be obtained from The Institute of Psychosexual Medicine (see Useful addresses, p. 331). Do send a stamped, addressed envelope.

SEXUALLY TRANSMITTED DISEASES

Sexually transmitted diseases (or venereal diseases, VD) are infections passed from one person to another during sexual intercourse, anal or oral sex. They carry the risk of serious damage to your reproductive organs, fertility and general health.

HIV (human immunodeficiency virus), the virus that's responsible for the illness AIDS (acquired immune deficiency syndrome), is the most serious sexually transmitted disease.

AIDS can kill and there is no cure for it. It is no longer an illness suffered only by gay men. The virus is spreading fast among heterosexual men and women. Pregnant women who have the HIV virus can pass it to their unborn child. A 1990 survey in London hospitals found that one in 500 babies tested positive for the HIV virus. The virus lives in the body fluids (blood, semen, vaginal secretions) of infected persons. The only protection against getting or giving the HIV virus is to practise safer sex. Safer sex is a code of sexual behaviour which aims to reduce the risk of becoming infected with HIV, or of passing it on. A condom prevents contact with the body fluids which carry HIV. Condoms additionally protect against other sexually transmitted diseases. They may also reduce the risk of cervical cancer, so it makes sense always to use one. Even if you are already using another contraceptive method (the pill for example), you should still use a condom to protect against infection. Using a spermicide as well may give extra protection against HIV.

Safer sex also means protecting yourself by changing sexual behaviour: restricting the number of your sexual partners, refusing casual sex, particularly in parts of the world where AIDS is a problem (for example, Central Africa, the West Indies, New York, California), and not indulging in high-risk sexual activities.

High-risk sexual activities are vaginal intercourse without a condom, anal intercourse (even with a condom), or any act which draws blood or causes semen or blood to enter the partner's body (oral sex, for example). There is no risk of contracting HIV from general body contact, stroking, caressing or body kissing.

If you think you could be infected with a sexually transmitted disease, it's important to seek your doctor's advice promptly.

Alternatively, get help from a sexually transmitted disease clinic – also known as a Genito Urinary Medicine or GUM clinic – at a hospital, where you will be treated completely confidentially.

Non-specific genital infection

This may cause a slight increase in vaginal discharge, but is often symptomless.

Treatment: Vaginal examination and swab taken for culture. A course of antibiotics is usually prescribed.

Trichomonal vaginitis

May cause thick, greenish-yellow vaginal discharge, vaginal irritation, pain on intercourse.

Treatment: Diagnosis is confirmed by taking a swab of the discharge. A course of anti-microbial drugs is normally prescribed.

Gonorrhoea

May be symptomless in women, or cause abnormal vaginal discharge and/or painful urination. Untreated infection can spread to womb and Fallopian tubes causing lower abdominal pain.

Treatment: Diagnosed by vaginal swab. Usually a course of antibiotics is given.

Syphilis

In its first stage a painless sore develops in the genital area or inside the vagina. This is highly infectious and disappears after a few weeks. In the second stage a rash appears all over the body, including the soles and palms. It does not itch.

Infectious wart-like lumps may appear around the anus and/or mouth.

Treatment: The disease is diagnosed by a blood test and samples taken from sores. Treatment is by a course of antibiotic injections followed by repeat blood tests for up to two years to check that the infection has not returned.

Herpes genitalis

Causes an intense itching in the genital area and a crop of small, painful blisters. These burst after twenty-four hours leaving small, painful ulcers which crust over. Glands in the groin may become swollen and painful. There may be raised temperature and a general feeling of being unwell.

Treatment: Your doctor may prescribe an antiviral drug or ointment to make blisters less sore and to speed healing. However, there is no complete cure and outbreaks do recur, although often they become milder over the years. Avoid sexual contact while there are blisters or sores to guard against infecting others.

Chlamydial infection

This is a very common microorganism which is responsible, in men, for non-specific urethritis (NSU), the most common sexually transmitted disease in the UK. Unfortunately in women the equivalent infection, non-specific genital infection (NSGI), is usually symptomless. It can however lead to infection of the Fallopian tubes, salpingitis (see Vaginal discharge, p. 184) which if left unchecked can cause infertility. If you have ever had any partners with NSU, or think you may have been infected with chlamydia, it is important to get checked.

Treatment: With antibiotic drugs, usually quick and successful. It is important for your partner to be treated also as the infection can ping-pong back and forth between you.

HIV

The human immunodeficiency virus is responsible for AIDS.

This is a disease which damages the immune system so that the sufferer cannot fight infection. A person becomes HIV-positive after being infected with the HIV virus during sexual or anal intercourse, or from contact with the blood or body fluids of an infected person. Being HIV-positive does not mean that a person will necessarily develop AIDS. Present estimates show that within ten years 50 per cent of HIV-positive people will go on to develop AIDS.

There are not normally any symptoms when a person becomes infected with HIV. The only way of telling if you have been infected is to take a blood test, which shows the presence of HIV antibodies in the blood.

Treatment: There is no cure for the HIV virus. Prevention is the only cure. This means practising safer sex, using a condom and avoiding coming into contact with the blood or body fluids of HIV-positive people. Intravenous drug-users who share needles, for example, are especially at risk. Advances in understanding have prolonged the life-expectancy of AIDS sufferers by treating the infections they are prone to. Much research is currently under way to improve treatments, but above all to try to develop a vaccine against the HIV virus.

VAGINAL BLEEDING, IRREGULAR

Bleeding between periods, as opposed to irregular periods (p. 174), especially if it causes pain, should always be investigated by a doctor. It may be a sign of a disorder that needs treatment.

Vaginal bleeding during pregnancy (p. 200) also requires investigation and should never be ignored.

Bleeding after intercourse

This can be a sign of an infection of the cervix, or more seriously, of abnormal or pre-cancerous cells which, if not treated, can develop into cancer of the cervix.

Treatment: Your doctor will undertake a vaginal examination and take a smear test. This will be sent for analysis to detect any abnormal cells. If such cells are found, you will probably be sent for further investigations such as a colposcopy (examination by a special microscope inserted into the vagina) to allow the doctor to take a closer look at the cervix, or a minor operation called a cone biopsy. During this, a sample of tissue is taken for analysis and examination.

Freezing and laser surgery are both highly successful treatments for abnormal cells of the cervix.

Bleeding after the menopause

This can be caused by a minor disorder, but may also be a symptom of a more serious cancer of the cervix or the uterus.

Treatment: Your doctor will undertake a vaginal examination and a smear test. Cancer of the cervix is treated by hysterectomy and/or radio- or chemotherapy.

Cancer of the uterus may require a hysterectomy and possibly radiotherapy and/or drug treatment.

Bleeding between periods, if you have an IUD or take the contraceptive pill

Both these methods of contraception may cause spotting or bleeding. This is not generally serious, but should be reported to a doctor.

Treatment: Your doctor may suggest an alternative method of contraception.

VAGINAL DISCHARGE

The vagina is usually kept moist and clean by a thin, whitish discharge. This normal discharge may increase or become clear or slippery in the middle of the menstrual cycle just before ovulation, during pregnancy, or during sexual arousal. Any discharge which is unusually profuse or offensive, especially if it causes vaginal itching or irritation, should be investigated by your doctor. Some sexually transmitted diseases can cause abnormal vaginal discharge and need prompt treatment.

Thick, white discharge

This is most often caused by vaginal thrush, a fungal infection that causes intense irritation. It can be a very persistent infection, recurring over and over again, especially after taking antibiotics, during pregnancy, or while taking the contraceptive pill.

Treatment: Your doctor will examine you and may take a swab of the discharge for analysis. He will probably prescribe a course of anti-fungal vaginal pessaries lasting around two weeks. He may prescribe cream for your partner's penis, to stop him re-infecting you. It is a good idea to abstain from intercourse while taking the treatment to prevent re-infection. If you take the contraceptive pill and regularly suffer from thrush, you may wish to change to another contraceptive method (see Contraception, p. 158).

Greenish-yellow, very smelly discharge with irritation

A forgotten tampon or diaphragm may cause a smelly discharge with irritation. Remove it immediately and consult your doctor if the discharge continues for more than twenty-four hours afterwards. More often, this type of discharge and irritation is caused by an infection by the trichomonal organism, which is sexually transmitted.

Treatment: A sample of discharge is usually taken for analysis. A course of anti-bacterial drugs is the usual treatment.

Abnormal discharge with pain in the lower abdomen and/or back/temperature/feeling generally unwell

This can be a sign of infection of the Fallopian tubes, sometimes called salpingitis. This is commonly caused by an infection spreading upward from the vagina, cervix or uterus. It can be due to infection from a sexually transmitted disease such as chlamydia or gonorrhoea (see Sexually transmitted diseases, p. 179); it may also follow childbirth, miscarriage or abortion. If salpingitis persists the infection may damage the insides of the Fallopian tubes and lead to infertility.

Treatment: Your doctor will undertake a vaginal examination and take a swab for analysis. He may prescribe painkillers. A course of antibiotics is the usual treatment to counter infection. In severe cases a short stay in hospital may be necessary.

PREGNANCY AND CHILDBIRTH

PREGNANCY AND CHILDBIRTH

Childbirth is safer than it's ever been. Thanks to better diet, improved living conditions, and effective medical care, your chances of having a happy, healthy pregnancy, and of delivering a beautiful baby, have never been better.

Ante-natal care and classes stress the importance of mothers-to-be looking after themselves during pregnancy. Current thinking is that there's a good deal to be gained from eating well, getting enough rest and gentle exercise, avoiding stress and smoking, and avoiding or limiting alcohol, even before you try to conceive. Certainly, once you're pregnant, taking these steps will help you make good progress and give your baby the best start in life.

The vast majority of pregnancies progress smoothly and without complication. Thanks to regular ante-natal checks, any potentially dangerous conditions such as high blood pressure are generally picked up and treated well before problems arise.

Pregnancy is not an illness, and in the middle months many women find that they feel fitter and more full of energy than at any other time in their lives. It does, however, bring with it a great many changes in a woman's body, some of which may seem alarming to a first-time mother, and many women do unfortunately suffer from discomforts such as backache and sickness. Occasionally, there are more serious symptoms which should be reported to your doctor at once.

The following chapter aims to help you understand some of the changes associated with pregnancy, and to decide when a symptom should be reported to your doctor.

ABDOMINAL PAIN

It's hardly surprising that many women experience abdominal pain and discomfort during pregnancy, considering the dramatic changes this part of the body in particular is going through. Abdominal pain during pregnancy is usually due to the pregnancy itself, but it can also be caused by any condition that gives pain when you are not pregnant (see Abdominal pain, p. 19).

The cause of pain associated with pregnancy may depend on how far advanced the pregnancy is. In the early weeks, sickness and nausea may cause general discomfort. Later on, pain can signal the beginning of labour.

Only a small minority of pains indicate a serious problem.

Abdominal pain with backache and bleeding can be a sign of miscarriage (see Vaginal bleeding, p. 200). Any severe pain that comes on suddenly, or any continuous severe pain, should be reported to your doctor.

Pain in early pregnancy

Pain in the upper abdomen or chest

This is likely to be due to heartburn. During pregnancy, increased hormone levels cause a relaxation of the body's ligaments. This is necessary for all the stretching that's required for a baby to be born. The valve between the stomach and the gullet (oesophagus) is affected, sometimes allowing the stomach's acid contents to burp back up into the oesophagus.

Treatment: Eat smaller, more frequent meals. Avoiding fried or spicy foods may help. Try drinking a glass of milk before bedtime and sleeping propped up on pillows. Ask your doctor's or midwife's advice before taking any indigestion remedies.

Lower abdominal pain like period pain
This is very common during early pregnancy. Provided there is no bleeding or other symptoms, there is no cause for concern.
   Treatment: A comforting hot-water bottle may help relieve discomfort.

Sharp, severe pain on one side
This type of pain, especially if followed by bleeding, can be an indication of ectopic pregnancy. This is when a fertilized egg implants in a Fallopian tube instead of in the womb. Urgent medical help is needed.
   Treatment: If your doctor suspects an ectopic pregnancy, he will refer you to hospital. An ultrasound scan (see Medical diagnostic tests, p. 308) can confirm the site of the fetus if you are more than six weeks pregnant. If an ectopic pregnancy is confirmed, an operation to end the pregnancy will be required.

Pain in later pregnancy

Aching, dragging pain in lower abdomen
This type of discomfort is very common. It can begin as early as sixteen weeks, although it's more common from around twenty-six weeks on. It's called round ligament pain, and is caused by the stretching of the ligaments that support the uterus. The pain may be worse when standing up after sitting for a while. There may be occasional sharp, stabbing pains.
   Treatment: There is no treatment for this type of pain. The only comfort is that it usually disappears by about thirty-two weeks.

Pelvic pain
Many women suffer from considerable pelvic pain and discomfort as their pregnancy advances. The trouble may start as early as thirty weeks, with a severe aching that gets worse towards the end of the day. This is caused by the gradual relaxation of the

ligaments that hold the bones of the pelvic girdle together. It is part of the body's preparation for childbirth.

From about thirty-six weeks, the baby's head may engage in the pelvis. Some women feel heaviness, aching or pain from the pressure, and may find it more difficult to walk. Pain may sometimes be felt in the groin or down the legs.

Treatment: There is no specific treatment for these types of pain, other than rest. Lying down for half an hour generally relieves some of the discomfort.

Painful or aching ribs

This is caused by the growing baby putting increasing pressure on the lower ribs. It may begin as early as thirty weeks, and can become quite severely painful later on. The pain is often worse on the right side as the uterus usually causes more pressure to the right.

Treatment: There is nothing that can be done for this pain. The only thing that relieves it is the birth of the baby, when it will disappear as if by magic.

Regular, cramping pains/low backache

These are both signs of the onset of labour. Other indications that labour has started include a 'show' of mucus (blood-stained or otherwise) from the vagina, or a loss of clear fluid if the waters break. If you suspect that your labour has started, call your doctor, midwife or maternity ward.

BACKACHE

This is unfortunately a very common problem. During pregnancy, increased hormone levels cause a relaxation of the body's ligaments. This is necessary for all the stretching that's required when a baby is born. These hormones act on the ligaments supporting the spinal column and pelvis. An alteration in the alignment and shape of the spine and pelvis, and tension in the muscles supporting them, results in the classic low backache of pregnancy which can, in some cases, become very painful.

Unfortunately, backache tends to become worse as the pregnancy progresses and the weight of the baby increases.

Treatment: The best treatment for backache is prevention.

Gentle exercise to improve posture and muscle-tone can be very beneficial. Yoga exercises for pregnancy and swimming are both excellent for preventing problems and also in helping to relieve pain. The following books are recommended reading for exercise during pregnancy:

Exercises for Childbirth, Barbara Dale and Johanna Roeber, Random Century, £5.95

Active Birth, Janet Balaskas, Unwin Paperbacks, £3.95

It's important to pay attention to posture. Try to stand upright with your weight evenly distributed, and when sitting ensure that the back has good support.

Low back pain and pain in buttocks

This is usually caused by a 'twist' in the sacro-iliac joint at the top of the buttocks. It can be very painful indeed and prevent walking in severe cases. Twisting movements such as turning over in bed or lying on your back make the pain worse.

Treatment: Physiotherapy or manipulation can sometimes relieve severe pain. Exercises as described above can help prevent the problem.

Backache with vaginal bleeding and/or cramping pains in lower abdomen

In early pregnancy, these symptoms can be a sign of miscarriage (see Vaginal bleeding, p. 200).

Backache with bleeding in late pregnancy can signal the

beginning of labour. If you suspect that you have started labour, call your doctor, midwife or labour ward for advice.

BREATHLESSNESS

The lungs have to work at a considerable disadvantage during the last three months of pregnancy, as the growing baby squeezes them up into a smaller and smaller space. Although the ribs push out to give a bit of compensating room, from about twenty-eight weeks onward you may find that you become breathless quite easily after only a little effort, such as walking up stairs. Giving up smoking (it's especially ill-advised to smoke during pregnancy) and avoiding excess weight gain can help prevent excessive shortness of breath.

Breathlessness before twenty-eight weeks, or breathlessness while resting, is not normal, and you should consult your doctor.

Treatment: Will depend on the cause of the problem.

CONSTIPATION

Constipation can be a problem for women who've not previously suffered from it. As with several other problems, the cause is often due to the general relaxation of the body's tissues because of the influence of changing hormone levels. The intestine may become over-relaxed and not be as efficient as usual at moving its contents along. Additionally, iron supplements given during pregnancy may cause constipation.

Treatment: Increasing fluid intake, stepping up the amount of fruit, vegetables and cereals you eat, and taking some gentle exercise, is usually enough to ease constipation. If you suspect that iron pills are contributing to the problem, speak to your doctor. He should be able to prescribe it in a different form.

Don't dose yourself with laxatives during pregnancy. If the

self-help measures described here don't work, see your doctor for advice.

CRAMP

Many women suffer from cramp in the calves, thighs or buttocks, and sometimes in the lower back. It is not a serious symptom but can sometimes be painful. Cramp often comes on towards the end of the day, or at night when the muscles are tired. It has been suggested that it may be due to calcium deficiency, but this hasn't been proved.

Treatment: Both during and in-between attacks, try to stretch the muscles which are cramping. A hot-water bottle can help the pain.

DEPRESSION AFTER CHILDBIRTH

As many as one in ten women receive medical treatment for depression after the birth of a baby. Doctors are undecided whether post-natal depression is caused by hormonal imbalance following childbirth, or by the pressures of coping with a small baby. Probably the truth is that depression results from a complex mixture of both, and that sleepless nights and physical exhaustion contribute their share also.

The 'baby blues' is the common name for the tearfulness and low spirits that most women suffer in the week following childbirth. This is probably due mainly to hormonal re-adjustment, and it usually passes quite quickly. Tiredness, irritability, weepiness, feelings of frustration, fears of not being able to cope, helplessness and anger, are also common and quite normal in the weeks and months after childbirth. It is, after all, a major life-event involving considerable upheaval and emotional turmoil.

There is quite a fine line between this type of normal upset feelings and those of true depression. If you are suffering from any of these emotions and are worried about it, if you feel apathetic towards your baby, or withdrawn, and as if everything is too much effort, you should seek your doctor's help. Also, the Association for Post-natal Illness can supply helpful pamphlets (see Useful addresses, p. 328).

Treatment: Your doctor will talk to you and assess your general health. He may prescribe anti-depressant drugs or refer you to a specialist for more assessment. You may be offered psychotherapy to help you cope with your feelings and fears. In cases of severe depression, hospital treatment can help.

FAINTING OR FEELING FAINT

Feeling faint (feeling light-headed or cold and clammy) is common during pregnancy, particularly in the first three months. It's caused by low blood pressure due to the general relaxation of muscles around the blood vessels, and to the increased demands of the uterus. When blood pressure falls below a certain level, the blood supply to the brain is reduced, causing faintness. Faintness is especially likely after standing for a long time, when getting up from sitting or lying down, or when going too long between meals. Although it's unpleasant, fainting does no harm to mother or baby in itself, although falling down can cause injuries.

Treatment: Avoid standing for long periods if possible. If you have to stand, move your legs and feet around to keep blood circulating. Get up slowly from a sitting or lying position.

Make sure you don't go too long without eating.

NAUSEA AND SICKNESS

Sickness and/or vomiting affects almost all women during the first three months of pregnancy. It is due to the dramatic rise in hormones in the blood. It may cause loss of appetite and even some weight loss in the first months. Fortunately, it usually fades gradually from about twelve weeks onwards.

If you suffer vomiting several times a day, you should consult your doctor. Otherwise, self-help measures can give some relief until the problem passes of its own accord.

Treatment: Try to eat frequent, small amounts of bland foods – biscuits, toast, milk, mashed potato, or any other foods that agree with you. Avoid fatty, highly spiced foods, and any foods or cooking-smells that make you feel nauseous. If cooking makes you feel sick, try to arrange for someone else to take over until you feel well again.

If you are sick in the morning, have a cup of tea and a biscuit before you get up. Keep calm; avoid rushing about and becoming over-tired. Rest as much as possible. Don't dose yourself with anti-sickness medicines without your doctor's permission. Perhaps surprisingly, research shows that mothers with pregnancy sickness have a more successful pregnancy overall, and with slightly larger babies, than those who don't. No one knows quite why.

Severe vomiting (hyperemesis) several times a day may be treated by your doctor with drugs. In a very few rare cases, where vomiting could prevent the baby receiving enough food, hospital treatment with fluids given by drip may be needed for a few days.

SKIN CHANGES

Pregnancy may affect the skin in several different ways because of changing hormone levels. Skin may become drier and itchy, or get oily and be more prone to spots. As the pregnancy progresses, stretch marks may develop on the abdomen or thighs as weight is gained.

Other changes may include an increase in pigmentation. The nipples may become darker, and you may notice a dark vertical line running down from your navel. Some women develop darker freckles if they have them already, or blotchy pigmentation on the face.

Treatment: Drier or more oily skin than normal should be treated as you would normally, either with a moisturizer or a slightly astringent lotion.

You cannot prevent stretch marks with any kind of creams or lotions, although these can be soothing if the skin is sore, dry or itchy. Stretch marks will usually fade gradually after delivery. The best way to prevent them is to avoid putting on excess weight.

Increased pigmentation on the face or other parts of the body usually fades gradually in the weeks after the baby is born.

SWOLLEN ANKLES

During pregnancy there is a tendency for the body to retain more water than normal. Part of the weight increase in pregnant women is due to water retention. A slight amount of swelling in the ankles and legs is normal, especially towards the end of the pregnancy, in hot weather, after standing for some hours, and towards the end of the day.

Considerable swelling of the ankles, swelling of the face and/or sudden weight gain, can all be symptoms of pre-eclampsia, which needs immediate treatment, since it can progress towards eclampsia, a dangerous condition of pregnancy. If you have any of these symptoms, or if when you press your swollen ankles a slight indentation remains, report to your doctor right away.

Treatment: Your doctor will take your blood pressure and a urine sample. If pre-eclampsia is diagnosed, you will need to rest and may be prescribed drugs to reduce blood pressure and fluid retention. Severe cases may need admission to hospital and/or early delivery of the baby.

TIREDNESS AND INSOMNIA

Tiredness is a very normal feature of pregnancy. From about the sixth to the fourteenth week, many women feel very tired during the day, and ready to fall into bed exhausted by early evening. This extreme tiredness fortunately passes, and during the second trimester (second three months) most women feel extremely well and full of energy.

Towards the end of pregnancy, tiredness due to lack of sleep often sets in again. It can become difficult to sleep soundly, and you may be disturbed several times a night – to visit the lavatory, because the baby's kicking disturbs you, because 'the bump' makes it difficult to lie comfortably, or because of backache, cramp, or anxiety about the birth which lies ahead.

Excessive tiredness, especially with feelings of weakness and breathlessness, can be due to anaemia, and it is important to have this treated before the baby is born.

Treatment: Excessive tiredness should be reported to your doctor.

If he suspects anaemia, he will take a blood test and, if necessary, treat you with iron supplements.

Getting adequate rest throughout pregnancy is important. Some women need as much as ten hours' sleep a night. If your nights are very disturbed, do everything you can to catch up on some rest during the daytime.

Eating a nutritious, well-balanced diet will ensure that the body's increased energy demands are met, and help avoid anaemia and the fatigue that comes from low blood sugar levels. Moderate exercise can, paradoxically, help overcome fatigue. Activities such as swimming, yoga and walking can be relaxing and encourage a good night's sleep.

VAGINAL BLEEDING

Vaginal bleeding can be a sign of miscarriage and should always
be reported to your doctor.

Painless vaginal bleeding in early pregnancy

Some spotting of blood in early pregnancy is quite common.

Provided that it is not accompanied by pain, it is usually no
cause for concern. Spotting often occurs around the time when
a period would normally be due and hormone levels are low. It
can also be caused by vaginal infections or by an erosion –
inflamed area – of the cervix.

Treatment: Report the spotting to your doctor. He may advise
resting until the spotting stops. If the pregnancy continues, there
is no increased risk to the baby.

Painless vaginal bleeding in the first half of pregnancy

If bleeding is not accompanied by pain it is usually described
as a 'threatened miscarriage'. Usually, the pregnancy continues
normally and there is no threat to the baby.

Treatment: Consult your doctor. He will probably advise rest
in bed. He may arrange an ultrasound scan (see Medical diagnostic tests, p. 308) to check that the pregnancy is progressing
normally.

Vaginal bleeding with backache and/or cramping pains

Bleeding with pain is usually a sign of miscarriage in early or mid-pregnancy.

Treatment: Consult your doctor immediately. He will probably arrange hospital admission. You will be given an ultrasound scan (see Medical diagnostic tests, p. 308) and possibly other tests. If a miscarriage is confirmed, you may be given a D & C (see Periods, p. 172) to remove the contents of the womb. Most women are able to conceive again successfully after a miscarriage and have a normal pregnancy.

Vaginal bleeding in later pregnancy

Vaginal bleeding in the later stages of pregnancy is called ante-partum (before birth) haemorrhage. It may have several causes. It can be due to partial separation of the placenta from the wall of the womb, to a low-lying placenta, or to abnormalities of the cervix. It may also be a sign that labour is beginning, especially if a plug of blood-stained mucus has been passed.

Treatment: Call your doctor at once. He is likely to arrange admission to hospital, where tests such as an ultrasound scan (see Medical diagnostic tests, p. 308) and the monitoring of the baby's heartbeat can be carried out. In cases of severe bleeding, the baby may need to be delivered early by Caesarean section or by inducing labour.

VAGINAL DISCHARGE

An increase in vaginal discharge is one of the earliest signs of pregnancy and is normal, provided that the discharge is not smelly or extremely profuse.

Any frothy, smelly or irritating discharge should be reported to your doctor. These can be symptoms of sexually transmitted diseases, some of which can affect your unborn baby, and which need treatment (see Sexually transmitted diseases, p. 179).

Throughout pregnancy, the acidity and sugar content of vaginal secretions change, making infection with the candida fungus (thrush) much more common. This infection causes a thick, curd-like discharge which is often very irritating. Consult your doctor.

Treatment: If your doctor confirms thrush infection, he will probably prescribe a course of anti-fungal pessaries or cream.

VARICOSE VEINS

An increase in the volume of blood circulating in the body during pregnancy, and pressure from the developing baby, put extra stress on the veins. The walls may stretch and pools of blood collect, causing varicose veins. These are most common in the legs, but can also affect veins in the lips of the vagina, where they are called vulval varicosities, and those in the anus, causing piles, or haemorrhoids.

Treatment: Vulval varicosities disappear after delivery; generally, piles shrink considerably or disappear completely.

Unfortunately, varicose veins in the legs can remain. Preventing them developing further as soon as they appear by exercising to improve circulation, resting often with the legs up during the day, and wearing support tights, is important. Surgical treatment to remove varicose veins, or injecting them with a substance that 'shrinks' them, may be suggested if they do not improve after childbirth.

BABIES AND CHILDREN

BABIES UNDER ONE

In many ways, parents are the real 'experts' when it comes to children's ailments. They know their child better than anyone else, and they shoulder the responsibility of deciding what action to take directly their child is unwell.

Yet with babies under one year, parents may find it difficult to judge when a child is ill, especially if it's their first. Perfectly normal, healthy little babies may suffer from sneezing and snuffling, changes in colour, inexplicable crying, rashes and spots. On the other hand, these symptoms can at times be signs of problems that need immediate medical attention.

So how can you tell when you should seek medical advice? We hope that the following chapter will help. Remember, above all, that you, better than anyone else, know what is 'normal' for your baby. If your baby is less than a year old, seems unwell to you, and you are worried, that's enough reason to pick up the telephone and speak to your doctor. Never be afraid to call or to go to the surgery straightaway if you think your baby is ill. Don't wait until the morning to see if things improve; in some cases small babies can become seriously ill very quickly if not treated. No one will ever think you foolish or fussy where the health of a baby is concerned.

Fortunately, the majority of babies' and children's illnesses are minor, but there are some signs you should never ignore. Seek medical help urgently if:

- The baby will not feed or take water and/or he is vomiting or has diarrhoea
- Breathing is noisy or abnormally fast, or the baby's breaths 'suck' in the lower chest.

- The baby has a fever. A temperature of over 39° C (102° F) needs medical attention
- The baby seems unusually drowsy, is hard to wake up or is irritable

BIRTHMARKS

This is a general term used to describe a wide range of skin marks or blemishes on newborn babies. Most babies have some kind of mark or blemish. Some are caused by pressure during the birth and will vanish within a week or so. Others are due either to abnormal blood vessels in the skin (red or purplish marks) or to uneven skin pigmentation (dark marks).

Bright-red, raised swelling

This is known as a strawberry naevus (capillary haemangioma). It can appear anywhere on the body and is not always visible at birth, but may show up shortly afterwards. These marks may get bigger for up to eighteen months, or they may start to shrink after the first six months. By the age of six years, however, nearly all of them have disappeared, leaving a fine, non-pigmented area of skin.

Treatment: Is not necessary or desirable, since interference may lead to scarring. Occasionally, a naevus is removed if it is near the eye and interferes with vision.

Flat red or purplish mark

This is known as a port wine stain (cavernous haemangioma). It can appear on any part of the body, but is most common on the face or neck. This birthmark does not disappear.

Treatment: Large or unsightly marks can be camouflaged with special cosmetics. Most plastic surgery clinics have trained cosmetic counsellors. Advances in plastic surgery techniques, and especially in the use of lasers, are offering better cosmetic results and the possibility of removing the marks in childhood.

Bluish, bruise-like marks on back or buttocks

These are known as Mongolian blue spots and are common among babies born to parents of African, Asian or Mediterranean descent. They disappear naturally by the time the child is two.
Treatment: No treatment is needed.

DIARRHOEA

If your baby is passing runny, watery motions more often than usual, he is suffering from diarrhoea. Extra sugar in fruit juice or sweet drinks can cause diarrhoea in babies; so can some syrupy medicines. If the baby has diarrhoea and a high temperature and/ or vomiting (see High temperature, p. 213, and Vomiting, p. 218), gastroenteritis, an infection of the digestive tract, is likely.

In this case, get your baby to the doctor immediately; don't wait until the morning to see if he's better. Small babies can become dehydrated very quickly, especially if they are vomiting as well.

Treatment: The baby needs to take extra fluids to make up for those lost. He must take several ounces of cooled boiled water or well-diluted fruit juice at least every two hours. The doctor may advise you to avoid formula milk and all solids for at least twenty-four hours, since these may make diarrhoea worse. If breastfeeding, give additional fluids. Rehydration sachets containing powdered glucose and mineral salts, which are made up with cooled boiled water, are sometimes prescribed.

EXCESSIVE CRYING

All babies cry; it is their only way of communicating physical discomfort or emotional distress. The difficulty for parents is in trying to decide how much crying is normal, and when the crying could be due to some definite problem that needs to be sorted out.

Crying with no obvious sign of illness or injury

If the baby is pacified by food or attention, it seems likely that it's not illness causing the crying. Here are some of the most usual reasons for crying in small babies:

Hunger
This is the most common cause of crying, and the most likely explanation for persistent crying in an otherwise well baby. Always offer a feed when your baby cries, even if it's been only a short time since the last one.

Lack of physical contact
Many small babies feel uncomfortable when deprived of physical contact. It's natural for them to feel most content when they are being cuddled or held. Picking up the baby and cuddling him against your shoulder so that his stomach and chest are pressed against your chest will almost always stop crying due to lack of 'contact comfort'. Walking with the baby held like this is especially soothing.

Babies can't be 'spoiled' by being held and cuddled like this. They don't cry deliberately to annoy you, and depriving them of attention makes them crave it more, not less. If your baby needs to be held a great deal, try using a carrying-sling to allow you to get on with everyday chores.

Tiredness
Some babies may become tired yet cannot relax enough to allow themselves to drop off to sleep. If your baby is otherwise well, and you have eliminated hunger and tummyache as possible causes, try soothing your baby to sleep by rocking, or offering the breast or a dummy for comfort. Rocking and sucking will often soothe a fretful baby to sleep.

Wind
Small babies often swallow air when they are feeding. The excess air can cause discomfort and crying if the baby is not 'burped'. Holding the baby upright on your lap or over your shoulder after feeding and gently patting the back for a few minutes can help to bring up wind and so avoid discomfort later on.

Being too hot or too cold
Feeling too hot or cold can make your baby cry – a baby's own temperature-regulating mechanism is inefficient in the first few months of life.

Sudden unusual crying, or persistent crying

If your baby is crying persistently, or if his crying sounds unusual to you, if he is not hungry or has refused food and/or he seems generally unwell, he may be suffering from an illness of some sort and you should seek your doctor's advice straightaway.

Minor illnesses include colic, teething, fever or a common cold (see High temperature, p. 212). More serious illnesses may include an infection, especially a middle-ear infection, which can be very painful and needs immediate treatment by a doctor. If you are concerned about persistent or unusual crying you should seek your doctor's advice straightaway.

FEEDING PROBLEMS

Concern about feeding is one of the most common worries for parents of babies and toddlers. Generally speaking, if the baby is gaining weight, is lively and seems well, it's pretty certain that he is getting enough to eat. However, poor feeding, constant hungry crying, faddy and difficult feeders, can be a cause of much misery for both parents and child. Breastfeeding mothers can have different worries and problems from those who bottle-feed. Feeding problems sometimes occur when progressing from one stage to another – during weaning, or in moving a baby from 'mush' on to lumpy or more solid foods.

Frequent feeding

Both breastfed and bottle-fed babies feed very often in the first few weeks of life, and this is quite normal. Breastfed babies may want to feed every two hours or more often, for half an hour or more. Bottle-fed babies may last for three hours. Most child-care experts now agree that babies should be fed 'on demand', that is, as often as they ask for food, and not be held to some pre-determined schedule. As babies grow older, they gradually begin to feed less often, and by about six months most babies are happy with around four feeds a day.

At some time between three and six months, though, a baby cannot drink enough milk at each feed to satisfy him for long. He may start to demand extra feeds again, becoming hungry quite shortly after having been fed. This is a sign that he needs to move on to some solid foods.

Reluctance to feed

A sudden reluctance to feed in a baby under six months can be a sign of illness. Call your doctor if the baby goes more than three hours over his normal feed time, or if he seems unusually drowsy.

Many babies lose interest halfway through a feed and fall asleep at the breast or bottle. This is usually a sign that they are content and full. There is no cause for concern, provided that the baby is gaining weight normally and does not seem unwell in any way.

Crying at feeds or after feeding

Breastfed babies sometimes cry or squirm immediately after starting to suck at the breast. This often happens when the mother's 'let down' reflex is delayed. The milk does not flow quickly enough for the hungry baby, and he becomes impatient and frustrated. Alternatively, the milk may flow too quickly and overwhelm him. Crying or squirming halfway through, or after, a feed in both breastfed or bottle-fed babies may be due to wind making the baby uncomfortable. If you lift him and 'burp' him, he may quite happily go back to breast or bottle and finish the feed.

Refusing foods

Suddenly refusing food can be a sign of illness (see Reluctance to feed, above). If you are sure that your baby is not unwell, he may simply not like what he is being offered. During weaning, babies often object to the texture of foods as much as to the flavour.

Foods that are too thick, and even the tiniest lumps, may be spat out at first. Begin weaning with very smooth and runny foods (about as thick as single cream) and very gradually introduce different tastes and a thicker consistency. If the baby rejects one food, try it again a day or so later. Babies' tastes seem to change from day to day. Be patient and continue to offer a variety of foods. Learning to eat is a big new experience for a small baby. He needs to be taught to enjoy different tastes and textures.

HIGH TEMPERATURE

The mechanism that lowers body temperature is immature in babies and children, with the result that they can develop a very high temperature alarmingly quickly in response to infection by a virus or bacteria.

Normal body temperature may range from 36° to 37° C (97° to 99° F).

Small variations are no cause for concern if the baby seems well. However, if he feels or looks hot, is sweating, irritable and/or seems generally unwell, and has a temperature of 38° C (100.4° F) or over, he has a fever, and you should take steps to lower his temperature (see below). High temperature in babies can trigger febrile convulsions (see p. 214). If a baby's temperature rises above 39° C (102° F) you should call your doctor at once. The easiest way to check a baby's temperature is by placing a thermometer under the arm for three minutes. Bear in mind, though, that this may give a slightly low reading. Taking the temperature rectally is most accurate.

Alternatively, temperature indicator strips that are placed on the child's forehead can be used. These are widely available at chemist's.

Reducing a child's temperature

A high temperature can trigger fever fits in babies and small children, so it's important to reduce it as quickly as possible.

Keep the room cool, below 21° C (70° F). Take off blankets and covers; leave only a sheet. Remove the baby's stretchsuit or pyjamas; a nappy and vest is enough. Sponge his face, neck, arms and legs with warm water and leave them to dry.

Repeat the sponging if the temperature has not come down within thirty minutes.

Children's paracetamol syrup safely reduces fever in babies. Give the correct dose for the age as stated on the bottle, and never more, or more often than allowed. Never give a child under twelve aspirin, unless professionally advised to do so.

High temperature with diarrhoea and/or vomiting

It's likely that your baby has gastroenteritis (see Diarrhoea, p. 207, and Vomiting, p. 218). You should call your doctor straightaway.

High temperature and unusually drowsy, hard to wake or irritable

These can be symptoms of meningitis, especially if the child has been vomiting too. Meningitis is a medical emergency and needs immediate treatment. Get your child to the doctor or to the hospital straightaway.

Treatment: If meningitis is suspected, a lumbar puncture will be performed (see Medical diagnostic tests, p. 306) to make a firm diagnosis.

There is no specific treatment for viral meningitis, from which nearly all children make a complete recovery. Bacterial meningitis is much more serious and can be fatal or cause disabilities as a result of brain injury. It is treated with antibiotics, usually by injection. The child may be kept in intensive care and be given fluids by drip.

High temperature with crying due to pain/ pulling or tugging at the ear

Middle-ear infections often cause high temperature in babies and can be extremely painful. They are especially likely after colds and nasal congestion. Bad infections can cause an ear perforation. This normally heals and hearing is not damaged.

Treatment: A course of antibiotics is normally prescribed. Some doctors will also prescribe a decongestant nosespray or drops. Children's paracetamol syrup can be give to ease pain and fever. If the infection has caused a perforation of the eardrum, this should be checked later on by the doctor. There is a very slight risk of lasting infection.

High temperature with fast breathing

A chest infection is possible, especially if the baby has recently had a cold.

Treatment: Antibiotics will probably be prescribed. Paracetamol syrup can be given to reduce fever. The baby will need to drink plenty of fluids. In severe cases, hospital admission may be necessary.

High temperature with spots or rash

See Common childhood infectious illnesses, p. 275.

High temperature with fits

Febrile convulsions, or fever fits, occur when a child's temperature rises above a certain point. The child's arms and legs shake uncontrollably, and he may go blue in the face. Usually, such fits are short and harmless, even if rather alarming for the parents.

Treatment: Lay the baby on his stomach over a pillow to stop him choking or harming himself. Remove any vomit from the mouth with a finger to stop it being inhaled. If the convulsion continues for more than a few minutes, go to hospital immediately. Even if your baby recovers quickly from a fit, always call your doctor so that the baby can be checked for an underlying disorder.

SKIN PROBLEMS

Small babies' skin is very sensitive and often prone to unexplained irritations and rashes. Usually these are nothing to worry about. If, however, an odd rash lasts for more than a day and/or the baby seems unwell, you should consult your doctor.

Nappy rash

Urine and faeces irritate a baby's skin if left in contact with it. Sore skin can allow infections from bacteria or from thrush (the candida fungus) to develop. The skin may become broken, inflamed and painful.

Treatment: Prevent nappy rash by keeping the baby's bottom as dry as possible with frequent nappy changes. Always change the nappy as soon as it is soiled with faeces. Wash and dry the nappy area thoroughly, and apply a little protective cream after every nappy change – too much may interfere with the absorbency of a disposable nappy. If the rash does not clear within a few days using simple measures, the baby may have thrush. In this case, the doctor will prescribe a cream for the problem.

Inflamed, scaly or blistery rash

Infantile eczema is a pink or red rash, dry and scaly to start with, which may become weepy and sore. It usually affects the hands and wrists, the creases of the arms, the ankles, and behind the knees. Eczema is an allergic reaction and often runs in families which may also be prone to hay fever and asthma. It is not contagious.

Treatment: With mild rashes, avoiding bathing liquids, soaps, lotions and baby wipes may be enough.

Brownish, crusty patches on the scalp

This minor and harmless condition is called cradle cap, and is common in small babies. Very occasionally, it can be a sign of another skin disease such as eczema, so ask your doctor's advice if it doesn't clear up with the simple measures given below.

Treatment: Firm but gentle washing with an ordinary baby shampoo, or one specially formulated for cradle cap, will normally clear mild cases.

Gentle rubbing with baby oil may remove thicker crusts.

Spots and rashes and/or blotches

If the baby is generally well and feeding, there is usually no cause to worry, provided that the problem disappears within a couple of days. If, however, the baby seems unwell, spots or rashes can be a sign of an infectious illness such as chickenpox (see Common childhood infectious illnesses, p. 275).

SLEEPING PROBLEMS

Waking regularly in the night for feeds is quite normal for babies of up to one year. Waking at night is not a sign of illness unless a baby who has slept well suddenly begins waking regularly, or seems distressed. The most usual reason for waking is hunger. Generally, a small baby will sleep again once fed.

As the baby becomes older, and the number of feeds he takes each day decreases, the intervals of sleep between feeds should gradually lengthen. Eventually, he should regularly sleep through the night, or at least until the early hours of the morning.

A newborn baby may sleep as much as twenty-two hours out of every twenty-four, but after four months or so babies begin to need less sleep.

From about six months, the average number of hours' sleep is thirteen, although individual babies may vary from as much as eighteen to as little as nine hours' sleep a day. Parents often expect babies to sleep more than they need, and perhaps invent a problem where none exists.

Until nine months or so, babies cannot deliberately keep themselves awake. Provided they are well-fed and comfortable, they will sleep when they need to and wake when they've had enough. A baby who sleeps a great deal during the day may not sleep as long at night, so it may pay to let him take fewer naps during the day. From around nine months, a baby becomes able to stay awake deliberately. Sleep problems often begin at this stage with babies who don't want to go to bed (see Sleep problems, p. 253).

If your baby wakes regularly at night and is not hungry, it's worth checking whether noise, cold or anxiety due to disruption of his normal routine may be causing the upset.

Otherwise, the need for comfort and the reassurance of your presence is probably the most likely reason for waking.

SLOW WEIGHT GAIN

Keeping a regular check on the weight gain of a baby is one of the best ways of being sure that he is making normal progress and developing well. For this reason, babies are weighed whenever they attend a baby clinic – and measured too, from time to time. It is a good idea to have your baby weighed regularly, weekly until about three months, fortnightly until six months, and then monthly until the age of a year, so that you can see how well he is doing.

At the clinic, the baby's weight, length and head circumference will be plotted on a graph each time he is weighed and measured. These graphs show the complete range of weights which are normal for babies from birth onwards. Each baby will progress at a rate which is normal for him. Some large birth-weight babies may slow down after a month or so, and stop growing as quickly.

Many small birth-weight babies have a great deal of catching up to do, and grow very quickly in the first few months.

Provided that the baby continues to gain weight at a rate which is normal for him, and within the normal range shown on the graph, all is well.

A baby that fails to gain weight, suddenly stops gaining or even loses weight, needs to be checked further. Slow weight gain may mean that the baby is not getting enough to eat, or may be a sign of illness.

TEETHING

A baby begins to cut its first teeth at around five months. The two bottom front teeth are usually the first to appear, followed by the two top ones. Usually, all the milk teeth are through by the age of three.

A teething baby will dribble a great deal, chew everything he can get into his mouth, and may be rather irritable because his inflamed gums are sore. However, teething cannot cause fever, vomiting, diarrhoea, loss of appetite or convulsions. If your baby seems ill, consult the doctor as you would normally do.

Dismissing such problems as 'teething' is potentially dangerous.

Treatment: Chewing a hard object, a teething-ring or piece of rusk, can help. Teething gels which soothe the gums can be bought from the chemist's, but their effect is short-lived.

VOMITING

Small babies bring up small amounts of milk after almost every feed because of wind. This is not vomiting, and is no cause for concern. Vomiting is the forceful 'throwing up' of the contents of the stomach. It can be caused by many minor upsets, and is usually nothing to worry about. However, if a baby is sick more than twice a day, it could be the sign of a potentially serious illness, and you should call your doctor right away.

Vomiting with diarrhoea

This is likely to be caused by an infection of the digestive tract, gastroenteritis (see Diarrhoea, p. 207). Small babies can lose a dangerous amount of body fluid quite rapidly when they have vomiting with diarrhoea, and there is a danger that they could become dehydrated. A baby who is not feeding should still take at least 500 mls (17 fl oz) of fluids a day given frequently in small amounts.

Vomiting with high temperature and/or unusually drowsy/reluctant to feed

These can be symptoms of meningitis, although something less serious is more likely (see High temperature, p. 212).

Vomiting following a bout of coughing

Whooping cough, a contagious infection caused by bacteria, causes children to vomit after a bout of coughing. Young babies may become very short of oxygen during a coughing fit. If your baby turns bluish during a coughing fit, or has trouble breathing, call your doctor or get him to hospital at once.

ONE YEAR ONWARDS

ABDOMINAL PAIN

'Tummyache' in a child is a very vague symptom and, because of this, and the fact that it can be due to so many different causes, both physical and emotional, it can be especially difficult to deal with.

'Tummyache' may mean nothing at all; it can also be a sign of a medical emergency such as appendicitis. Parents have the tricky job of deciding when there's no cause for concern and when a doctor's advice is needed. You should always call a doctor if:

- the child is in severe pain
- the pain has lasted for more than six hours
- the child is vomiting greenish-yellow matter
- vomiting does not relieve the pain within three hours

Children under two are unlikely to complain of tummyache. They find it difficult to pinpoint where a pain is coming from. Be especially vigilant, therefore, with young children. If a young child lies curled up because of pain, or walks bent up in pain, call the doctor at once.

Pain with vomiting

Gastroenteritis (infection of the digestive tract) is the most probable cause of pain with vomiting, although there is also the possibility that this could be an early sign of appendicitis (see Vomiting, p. 270).

Treatment: If after vomiting the pain continues for more than three hours, get your child to the doctor immediately. Otherwise, treat as for gastroenteritis (see Diarrhoea, p. 233). Give the child only plain water to drink, little and often, and avoid solid foods for the next twenty-four hours, gradually introducing them again over the next few days. A well-wrapped hot-water bottle held to the tummy can help soothe the discomfort.

Pain with vomiting of greenish-yellow matter

An obstruction of the intestines or appendicitis is possible (see Vomiting, p. 269). This is a medical emergency, and you should get help immediately.

Treatment: Don't give your child anything to eat or drink until he sees a doctor. The child will probably be admitted to hospital for medical tests. If an obstruction is found, it will probably need to be treated by surgery.

Pain and tenderness

A pain that starts around the tummy-button and moves down towards the lower right groin is very typical of appendicitis. If the tummy is also very tender and/or the child is vomiting or unable to stand up straight, this is a medical emergency and you should get help immediately.

Treatment: Give the child nothing to eat or drink; only a well-wrapped hot-water bottle, held to the tummy, to ease the pain. If appendicitis is diagnosed after investigation in hospital, surgery is likely in order to remove the inflamed appendix.

Pain with fever and/or pain on urinating/urgency to urinate/bedwetting

An infection of the urinary tract caused by bacteria from the bowel is a possibility (see Urinary problems, p. 268). This is more likely in girls.

Treatment: Consult your doctor. A sample of urine will probably be taken for analysis. If infection is found, a course of antibiotics is the usual treatment.

Pain with sore throat and/or cold

Many feverish illnesses, such as sore throat, cold or an ear infection, may cause a small child to complain of mild tummyache. This is because in children the lymph glands in the abdomen swell as a result of infection, which is thought to be the cause of discomfort.

Treatment: Treat a cold (see Colds, p. 227) or sore throat in the usual way. If you suspect an ear infection, take the child to the doctor, who will probably prescribe antibiotics.

Recurrent tummyaches

Many children suffer regular bouts of tummyache with no apparent cause. It's possible that anxiety or tension may be to blame, although this is not always obvious.

Treatment: Have the child checked by the doctor just to rule out any physical cause. Try to establish if there is any pattern to the attacks, and so discover if any particular anxiety is causing them.

Treat the child sympathetically; whatever the reason for his pain, it still hurts. Resting in bed with a well-wrapped hot-water bottle and plenty of warm drinks can be soothing.

ABNORMAL-LOOKING FAECES

Changes in the appearance of faeces are nearly always due to a change in diet. Very occasionally, they may be a sign of an underlying problem that needs investigation.

Very pale faeces

Some forms of gastroenteritis (see Diarrhoea, p. 233, and Vomiting, p. 269) cause children (and adults) to pass unusually pale faeces for a few days. If your child has recently recovered from an illness such as this, there is no cause for concern. Consult your doctor if things aren't back to normal within a week.

Treatment: None is usually necessary.

Very pale, foul-smelling faeces

Sometimes a failure to digest fats properly can cause very foul-smelling faeces that float. See your doctor.

Treatment: Blood tests and tests on faecal matter will probably be arranged. Treatment will depend on the cause of the problem.

Blood in faeces

It is very unusual for children to pass blood in their faeces.

Any slight streaks of blood on the surface of the faeces are generally due to a small tear in the anus caused by constipation (see Constipation, p. 229). Bloody diarrhoea is caused either by dysentery (a serious infection of the digestive tract) or by an inflammation of the intestines. Both conditions are serious and need immediate medical treatment.

Treatment: Depends on the cause of the problem.

ACHING OR PAINFUL JOINTS

Painful joints, particularly those in the arms and legs, are nearly always caused by accidental strain or injury (see Injured arm or leg, p. 251), or are associated with a viral infection like flu.

However, there is a small chance that such pains could be caused by inflammation or infection in the joint or, very rarely, by a form of juvenile arthritis.

Pain following injury/child unable to move the painful joint

A fracture or dislocation is a possibility (see Injured arm or leg, p. 251).

Painful, swollen, hot or red joint

Inflammation of the joint due to infection is a possibility.

Treatment: Any painful, swollen joint should be examined by the doctor immediately. Infection can inflict quite rapid damage. Blood tests and possibly tests on a sample of fluid drawn from the joint may be necessary to confirm an infection. If an infection is found, antibiotics will probably be prescribed. Anti-inflammatory drugs and painkillers may also be necessary.

Painful joints with headache/cough/sore throat

A viral infection such as flu is the most likely cause.

Treatment: Keep the child warm and comfortable in bed with plenty of fluids and paracetamol syrup to relieve the pain. See your doctor if the joint pain becomes severe or does not improve within twenty-four hours.

Joint pain and stiffness and/or high temperature/ rash/swollen glands/abdominal pain

These are symptoms of juvenile arthritis, of which there are several types. Such symptoms should always be brought to your doctor's attention.

Treatment: Diagnosis of juvenile arthritis is not always easy.

Blood tests and X-rays are undertaken, and it may be necessary to watch the progress of the illness for a few weeks to rule out other possibilities. If the illness is confirmed, anti-inflammatory drugs and painkillers may be prescribed. Light splints may be used to rest the inflamed joints. Following this, physiotherapy is usually necessary to keep the joints mobile and strong. In most children, the arthritis gradually disappears after a few years, inflicting no permanent damage.

BEDWETTING

Bedwetting (enuresis) is usual until three years, common until five, and by no means rare even at the age of seven and above. A child cannot stay dry at night, however much he wants to, until his body is mature enough to let him. Being able to control the bladder at night, and recognize the signals that indicate that it is full, is a process of physical maturity.

Bedwetting can often result from expecting a child to stay dry at night before he is able to. Many children need nappies at night well past their third birthday. Boys seem to be slower to develop good bladder control than girls. If your child needs to urinate every couple of hours during the day, and has a wet nappy each morning, then he is not ready to stay dry at night.

Helping your child to stay dry at night

Learning to stay dry at night is a gradual process for most children. Minimize the inconvenience of wet beds by using a plastic sheet. Most experts don't advise keeping an older child in nappies. Nappies are for wetting. You need to encourage your child to respond to the signals that tell him that his bladder is full and get up, or call you to ask for the potty.

Keep a potty close at hand in the child's room so that he can get up and use it if he feels the need. If a child wakes up in the night to use the potty, this is a good sign. It means control is coming. Try to stay calm about accidents, however inconvenient they are. Adding anxiety to the bedwetting problem doesn't help.

Some parents restrict drinks last thing at night. This is not a good idea. Your child will then probably wake because he is thirsty. Others lift a child out of bed last thing at night to 'pot' him. Again, this may be counter-productive, because you are then encouraging a child to pee while half-asleep, the very thing you wish him to grow out of.

Treatment for bedwetting is rarely advised in children under six. For those over this age, the most effective method seems to be an enuretic alarm, which wakes the child when the bed become damp. Over time, most children learn to wake to the sensations of a full bladder without the help of an alarm.

Sudden bedwetting after a child has been dry for months

Episodes of bedwetting can often occur as a result of stress in a child's life. Starting school, the arrival of a new baby, or the parents' divorce, may all cause upset and result in accidents at night. Try not to make a fuss about the problem if the child is already anxious; it will not help. Also, avoid embarrassing him about the problem.

Occasionally, a urinary tract infection or other medical conditions such as diabetes may cause a recurrence of bedwetting.

If a normally dry child suddenly begins bedwetting, it is worth checking with your doctor to rule out such possibilities.

COLDS

A runny or blocked nose, possibly a cough and/or sore throat, are all symptoms of the common cold. Colds are caused by a viral infection of the nose and throat, and there is very little you can do to prevent your children catching them. There's never been any proof that taking extra vitamins or any other type of remedy can prevent us catching colds. On the other hand, children who eat well and are generally healthy may have more resistance to infection.

Babies are especially prone to colds and respiratory infections. Later on, coming into contact with lots of children when starting school or playgroup often dramatically increases the number of colds a child gets – as many as ten a year is normal. It takes several years for children to build some immunity to the many different cold viruses they are exposed to.

Colds in themselves are not dangerous, although they can make a child miserable, and a blocked and runny nose usually upsets a baby who may have trouble feeding because he needs to breathe through his nose when he sucks.

Colds aren't caused by getting wet feet, sitting in draughts, or going out without a coat on, although lowering the body temperature drastically might lessen a child's resistance to infection if he already has one.

Children often develop a temperature or even vomit at the beginning of a cold, but after this it doesn't usually make them ill; just irritable. Occasionally, a cold may pave the way for a secondary bacterial infection such as an ear infection, bronchitis or pneumonia. If a child develops a temperature, a thick, greenish nasal discharge, wheezy cough or sore throat, consult your doctor.

Treatment: There is no specific treatment for the common cold other than offering a child plenty of fluids and keeping him warm and comfortable in bed if he feels very unwell. Try to encourage your child to blow his nose to prevent build-up of mucus. A baby may need nosedrops from the doctor if a blocked nose is stopping him from feeding. These should be used sparingly and strictly as prescribed. Over-use may make the problem worse.

The doctor cannot prescribe anything for the cold virus, but if a secondary bacterial infection takes hold, a course of antibiotics is sometimes prescribed.

CONFUSION

If a child talks nonsense, appears dazed or confused, and is drowsy, dizzy or sick, you should get medical help.

Confusion with dizziness and/or vomiting/ headache/visual disturbance/odd-looking pupils after a head injury

Occasionally, blood vessels inside the brain are damaged following a blow to the head or a severe shaking. Slow bleeding into the brain may occur some time after the injury. If a child develops a headache (see Headache, p. 245), becomes dizzy, sick, can't see, or the pupils of his eyes look odd, this is a medical emergency.

Call an ambulance or get the child to hospital immediately.

Treatment: The child will probably be given a head X-ray and/ or CAT scan (see Medical diagnostic tests, pp. 309 and 303) to check for damage to the brain or skull. Surgery may be necessary.

Confusion with high temperature

A temperature over 39° C (102° F) can cause delirium and/or convulsions in children (see High temperature, p. 247). Call the doctor at once.

Treatment: Try to bring down the child's temperature (see p. 212) while you wait for medical help.

Confusion with headache/vomiting/stiff neck

These can all be symptoms of meningitis (see Headache, p. 246). See your doctor at once.

Confusion with moments of 'blankness' or loss of consciousness/twitching and jerking

See Fits, p. 239.

CONSTIPATION

Children vary considerably in how often they have a bowel motion.

Some may open their bowels several times a day, while for others once every two days is normal. Variations in usual bowel habit are quite normal too. A change in diet, or an illness which causes vomiting or loss of fluid from sweating, is enough to upset the normal routine. Sometimes anxiety about using the lavatory, when starting school, or going on holiday, for example, may make a child resist the urge to defecate. This in turn leads to hard motions which may be difficult or painful to pass, making him reluctant to defecate. A vicious circle can easily be set up.

Sometimes a small tear in the lining of the anus, an anal fissure, may cause pain on defecation, and possibly a small amount of blood. This too can make a child reluctant to use the lavatory.

Only if a child often has hard, infrequent motions which are difficult to pass is he said to be truly constipated.

Treatment: Adjustments to diet are usually enough to correct constipation.

Ensure that your child drinks enough fluids and that fresh fruit, vegetables and cereals form a good part of his diet, providing plenty of dietary fibre.

If you think he may be anxious about using the toilet, talk the problem through with him. Try to encourage a relaxed attitude, and explain that it's important never to resist the urge to defecate.

It's unwise to give children laxatives, except on your doctor's advice. These can set up bad bowel habits and make the problem of constipation worse, not better, in the long run.

COUGHING

Coughing is a normal reaction to irritation or congestion in the throat or lungs. It's the body's way of clearing mucus from the airways. Usually, coughing is caused by minor infections of the nose and throat. Occasionally, though, it may be a symptom of a more serious illness. You should get medical advice if:

- the cough causes rapid or noisy breathing (see Unusual breathing, p. 266)
- the cough causes pain in the chest
- green, yellow or blood-stained mucus is coughed up
- the cough lasts for more than ten days
- your child has choked on something which could have been inhaled into the lungs (see Essential first aid, choking, p. 290)

Uncontrollable bouts of coughing with noisy intake of breath and/or high temperature/ runny nose/vomiting

These are symptoms of whooping cough, pertussis, a highly contagious bacterial infection. Usually, sneezing and a runny nose come before the cough develops, and you may think that your child is starting a cold.

Typically, the cough begins at night in the early stages of the illness, and later becomes worse by day. As the illness progresses, bouts of coughing may be so violent and prolonged that they make the child vomit afterwards.

The illness may last as long as six weeks, and unfortunately it tends to recur. It is most dangerous in babies under a year who can be deprived of oxygen during coughing bouts, resulting occasionally in brain damage or even death.

Treatment: See your doctor. In some cases antibiotics can reduce the severity of symptoms if the illness is diagnosed early enough. A child with whooping cough needs careful nursing. He needs small, light meals after vomiting to prevent weight loss, plenty of fluids, and considerable comfort and affection during a coughing bout, which can be very frightening. Babies or small children with whooping cough may need hospital admission. A course of immunization starting at two months prevents the disease (see Immunization, p. 323).

Coughing with runny nose and/or high temperature/rash

Measles (see Common childhood infectious illnesses, p. 276) often starts with coughing, a runny nose and high temperature. The distinctive rash usually appears a few days later.

Treatment: There is no specific treatment for measles other than keeping the child comfortable in bed and keeping his temperature down (see High temperature, p. 212).

Cough with high temperature

Viral infections such as influenza are often preceded by a cough and a raised temperature.

Treatment: Keep your child resting comfortably in bed and

drinking plenty of fluids. There's no need to consult a doctor unless the symptoms become worse, the child has trouble breathing, develops a rash, or you are worried.

Cough with runny or blocked nose

The common cold often produces a cough which is the body's reaction to mucus dripping down the back of the throat.
   Treatment: See Colds, p. 227.

DEAFNESS

There are two main types of deafness. The first, usually present from birth, is caused by a problem in the inner ear, or in the nerve leading from the ear to the brain. It's most commonly caused by a family history of deafness, or by the mother getting German measles while pregnant. The second type is usually due to an inflammation, a blockage, or to damage to the middle ear, which stops sound getting to the inner ear.

Babies are routinely checked for hearing at birth, and then at developmental checks at around eight months, eighteen months, and three years. However, deafness can sometimes be overlooked in an older child, or can develop between these checks and not be spotted. It's important that deafness in babies and children is diagnosed and treated early. Those whose hearing is impaired will be held back in learning to speak, often at a crucial stage of development, and in other learning skills.

If you're concerned that your baby is not responding to sounds well, or you feel that he is slow in learning to speak, or an older child is falling behind at school, asks you to repeat things often and/or seems to need the television turned up very loud, and you're worried about his hearing, you should take him to the doctor directly.

Treatment: The doctor will examine your child's ears. If he finds infection or inflammation, a course of antibiotics will generally be prescribed. Ear infections following colds can sometimes cause temporary loss of hearing by blocking the eustachian tube, which runs between the middle ear and the back of the throat. Wax may also block the ear canal in the older child or teenager. If this is found, it can be softened by using eardrops and/or syringed out by a doctor or nurse.

Frequent infections or irritants which cause inflammation can block the eustachian tube and cause an accumulation of fluid in the middle ear, a condition known as glue ear. If antibiotics fail to clear this up, it can be treated by a small operation under general anaesthetic, a myringotomy. The fluid is drained and a small plastic tube, a grommet, is inserted into the eardrum. The grommet allows the fluid to drain and the ear to return to normal. It stays in place for about six months before it usually drops out naturally, by which time hearing is normally restored.

If congenital deafness is suspected, a full range of hearing tests will be arranged. Following the results, the child will normally be helped with hearing aids and assistance from a trained therapist.

DIARRHOEA

The most common reason for diarrhoea is an infection of the digestive tract, gastroenteritis (see Vomiting, p. 270). In older children, unlike babies, this is seldom any cause for concern. However, you should consult your doctor if the child:

- has stomach pain for longer than six hours
- vomits repeatedly for more than twelve hours
- refuses drinks
- doesn't pass urine for over six hours
- is very drowsy or has sunken eyes

Excitement, an emotional upset, or a change in diet can sometimes cause diarrhoea. Constipation occasionally causes hard

motions to block the rectum partially, allowing liquid matter to
leak past.

Treatment: If you suspect that your child has gastroenteritis,
give no solids, only plenty of clear fluids (water, diluted fruit
juice, clear soups) for the first day. Gradually introduce solids
over the next four days, starting with mashed or pureed vegetables or fruits (mashed potato or stewed apple is ideal). Make
sure that you wash your hands thoroughly before preparing food
and after using the lavatory to guard against spreading infection.
Tell the child to do the same. Don't share flannels or towels.

DROWSINESS

Drowsiness is most often the result of not enough sleep, or an
exceptionally late or disturbed night. A child who is coming down
with a cold or flu may also feel tired and sleepy. However,
unusual or unexplained drowsiness can be a symptom of serious
illness and you should never ignore it.

Drowsiness with high temperature and/or vomiting/headache/stiff neck

These are all symptoms of meningitis (see Headache, p. 246).
This is a serious illness and needs immediate medical attention.
See your doctor at once, or take the child straight to hospital.

Drowsiness following a fall or blow to the head

This can be a symptom of a serious head injury which is a medical
emergency (see Confusion, p. 228). Call an ambulance or get
the child to hospital at once.

Drowsiness with rash

An infectious illness is a possibility (see Common childhood infectious illnesses, p. 275).

Drowsiness with unusual thirst/passing large amounts of urine/bedwetting/loss of weight/feeling tired all the time

These are all symptoms of diabetes, a disease caused by the body not producing enough insulin. Insulin is a hormone made by the pancreas which allows sugars in food to be converted into energy. If the pancreas fails, the level of sugar (glucose) in the child's blood and urine rises.

Treatment: Consult your doctor if your child develops any of these symptoms. A simple blood and urine test will show up abnormal levels of glucose. If the results are positive, the child will be referred to a specialist. Treatment to replace missing insulin is usually by injection or tablet. Diet must be carefully monitored.

Drowsiness with headache and/or red eyes/loss of appetite/constant tiredness/difficulty getting up in morning/poor or unusual behaviour

In older children the possibility of alcohol, drug or solvent abuse should be considered. Could your child have been drinking, or had access to drugs prescribed for an adult (e.g. tranquillizers) or to illegal drugs? These worrying possibilities should be considered, especially if there have been complaints from the child's school about behaviour or performance. If you suspect any such difficulties, you should confront your child with your fears immediately. Seek advice from your doctor or the child's school if you need help, information, or support with the problem.

EARACHE

Ear infections are very common in babies and young children, and can be very painful and distressing. If a baby has a high temperature (see Babies under one, high temperature, p. 213), tugs at his ear, cries continually, yells in pain, or begins waking and crying at night, suspect earache. Most ear problems in babies and young children are caused by infections, often stemming from colds and coughs.

Some small children manage to poke small pieces of toys or beads into their ears, which set up inflammation and infection, so consider this possibility also.

Treatment: The doctor will examine the child's ears and, if he finds inflammation, will probably prescribe a course of antibiotics. These may take up to twenty-four hours to work. In the meantime, children's paracetamol syrup taken in the recommended dosage will help relieve the pain. Should the cause of the problem be a foreign body in the ear, this must of course be removed by the doctor or nurse, often by syringing the ear.

EYE PROBLEMS

Most soreness, itching and redness of the eyes or eyelids is caused by infection or irritation. Other common problems include a foreign body stuck in the eye and injury to the eye.

Sticky discharge from eye/white of eye looks red/eye watery and sore

Conjunctivitis, an inflammation of the membrane covering the surface of the eye and inside eyelids, can cause these types of symptom. It is usually the result of a bacterial or viral infection.

Treatment: The doctor will probably prescribe antibiotic eyedrops or ointment. Bathe the eyelids gently with cooled boiled water to remove the discharge, making sure that you use a fresh piece of cotton wool each time you wipe. This avoids spreading the infection. Don't share towels or face-flannels with other family members for the same reason.

Sticky discharge from eye/watery eye/sore eyelid in babies

About 2 per cent of babies are born with a blocked tear duct. This stops the tears draining away, and the eye can become infected and sticky. The eyelids may get stuck together, especially when the baby's been sleeping.

Treatment: Bathe the lids of the infected eye gently with cooled boiled water and sterile cotton wool. Use a fresh piece for each wipe. The doctor may prescribe antibiotic eyedrops or ointment. He will also show you how to massage the tear duct gently to clear the blockage. This problem usually corrects itself by the time the baby is one year old. If it persists, a simple operation can unblock the tear duct.

Itchy, red eyelids

A generalized inflammation, blepharitis, can cause sore, itchy or scaly eyelids and/or swollen, sore rims around the eyes.

Treatment: Antibiotic eyedrops or cream may be prescribed to clear the infection. Try to stop the child rubbing his eyes.

Red lump on the lid

Styes are caused by an infection at the root of an eyelash.

Treatment: Generally, styes burst naturally, releasing pus, or else dry up of their own accord. Wipe away any discharge with a piece of cotton wool dipped in cooled boiled water. Use a fresh piece each time you wipe to avoid spreading infection. Consult your doctor if the stye doesn't heal after about a week.

Something stuck in eye

Specks of dirt or small particles on the white of the eye or inside the lids may be safely removed using the moistened corner of a handkerchief. Never try to remove anything embedded in the eye or on the membrane – the cornea – over the central part of the eye (the iris and pupil). In this case cover the eye with a clean handkerchief, the eyelid closed, and seek medical help at once.

Chemicals in the eye

Any chemicals splashed in the eye that cause pain and soreness should be immediately flushed out with lots of cold water. Hold the child's head sideways over a sink with the affected eye downwards. Hold the eyelids open and pour water over the eye until the substance has been flushed out. Then seek medical help.

Cuts or blows to the eye or eyelid

Any such injury requires urgent action. Cover the injured eye gently with a clean pad and hold in place with a bandage or scarf. Get the child to the nearest hospital casualty department as quickly as possible.

FAINTING

Fainting, a temporary loss of consciousness, is not usually any cause for concern in an otherwise well child. It's caused by a sudden drop in blood pressure brought on by a fright, anxiety, or by being hungry. Often a child will go white or complain of feeling dizzy before a faint.

Treatment: If the child remains unconscious for more than a minute, seems to have trouble breathing, or is shaking while unconscious (see Fits, below), get medical help. Otherwise, lie the child out flat on the floor with the legs raised if this is possible, or sit him down with his head between his knees. Loosen any tight clothes and make sure that there's plenty of fresh air. When the child comes round, offer a sweet drink and a small snack.

If your child often faints, it's probably wise to consult a doctor.

FITS

Fits, or convulsions, are quite common during childhood. One child in twenty will suffer at least one episode of loss of consciousness with jerking or twitching of the arms, legs or whole body. Fits are extremely distressing to witness, but are usually not harmful unless they happen often or are prolonged.

Children's fits are often triggered by a high temperature due to an infection (see High temperature, p. 247, and Babies under one, high temperature, p. 212). In babies and children, the mechanism for lowering temperature is immature and a very high temperature can develop alarmingly quickly. Fever fits, often called febrile convulsions, tend to run in families, and are frequently outgrown by the time the child is five.

Fits may also be caused by abnormal electrical activity in the brain. Such fits, if they happen repeatedly, are usually diagnosed as epilepsy. Epileptic fits are more common in children than in adults, although it's not known why. Many children 'grow out' of epilepsy as they become older.

Loss of consciousness with high temperature

See High temperature, p. 247, and Babies under one, high temperature, p. 212.

Sudden loss of consciousness/falling to the ground/body rigid or jerking and twitching

The type of epileptic fit which causes a child to fall down is known as grand mal. There is a danger that a child might injure himself during the fall. He may also vomit, pass urine, or have a temporary memory loss on regaining consciousness.

Treatment: During an attack, the priority is to prevent the child injuring himself. Place the child on his stomach with head to one side. Move any nearby dangerous objects away. Don't try to restrain the child or to force anything into his mouth.

If loss of consciousness lasts longer than ten minutes, get medical help straightaway. Otherwise, allow the child to sleep naturally when the convulsions have stopped. Always report such fits to the doctor. If he suspects epilepsy, the child will probably be referred to a specialist for diagnosis and treatment.

An EEG (see Medical diagnostic tests, p. 304) may be performed. Anti-convulsive drugs may be prescribed to control the convulsions.

Momentary loss of consciousness/periods of 'blankness'/glazed eyes/twitching face or limbs

Momentary loss of consciousness lasting only ten to fifteen seconds, when the child seems 'vacant' but doesn't fall down, can be a sign of a milder form of epilepsy called petit mal.

Treatment: No special treatment is needed during an attack. If the fits are frequent, the doctor will probably refer the child to a specialist. An EEG (see Medical diagnostic tests, p. 304) will probably be performed to confirm the diagnosis. Anti-convulsive drugs may be prescribed. Children often grow out of petit mal attacks by the time they are teenagers.

GENITAL PROBLEMS

Boys

Pain or swelling of the scrotum (the sac that supports the testes) can be caused either by injury or by infection. Severe pain in this region should always be treated as a medical emergency, and the child should be taken to hospital immediately.

Painful swelling in the scrotum following injury
If the pain does not subside quickly, take the child to hospital.

There may be internal damage to the testes which needs immediate attention.

Treatment: The boy should be carefully examined. Sometimes no treatment is needed, but in certain cases an operation to repair damage may be necessary.

Painful swelling of the scrotum following mumps
Inflammation of the testes following mumps (orchitis) is a possibility in an older boy; it is rare in young children.

Treatment: Consult your doctor. If orchitis is confirmed, he will possibly prescribe an anti-inflammatory drug.

Unexplained pain and swelling/possible nausea and vomiting
The twisting of the testicle out of its normal position (torsion of the testicle) is a possibility. This can occur without any apparent cause. It can be extremely painful.

Treatment: Torsion cuts off the blood supply to the testicle and immediate action is required to prevent permanent damage. Rush the child to hospital if torsion is suspected. If confirmed, a doctor may gently try to untwist the testicle manually, but if this fails immediate surgery will be necessary.

Painless swelling inside the scrotum

This could be caused by a discrete cyst, by a large accumulation of fluid (a hydrocele), or by an inguinal hernia, caused when part of the abdominal contents pushes through a weak part of the abdominal wall.

Treatment: Consult your doctor. A cyst or hydrocele (not common in childhood) will usually be left alone, or drained by a syringe, or removed.

Hernia is treated by a repair operation.

Soreness or swelling of tip of penis

A bacterial infection of the foreskin (balanitis) is likely. This is especially common in babies. A baby may cry when passing urine and the penis may become red and swollen with a slight discharge.

Treatment: Consult a doctor who will probably prescribe a soothing antibiotic cream. Take extra care by regular washing of the baby's bottom and penis, and urge an older child to do the same.

Discharge from the penis

Occasionally small children may push objects into the penis which set up infection if they are not expelled.

Treatment: Consult a doctor. The object may need to be removed by a minor operation.

Girls

Itching and inflammation of the vulva (the external genital area) causing pain on urination may be the result of an infection or an irritation from soaps or perfumed toiletries. Unusual vaginal discharge may be caused by a number of factors.

Itching or sore genital area

May be caused by irritation from perfumed toiletries.

Occasionally such infection may be due to urinary tract infection (see Urinary problems, p. 268) or to threadworms.

Treatment: Try self-help measures first. Wash the genital area once a day with plain warm water only. Use no talcs or toiletries. An unperfumed barrier cream, such as petroleum jelly, on the sore area can help to prevent further irritation. The child should wear only cotton underpants, changed daily.

If irritation persists, consult your doctor. He may take a urine sample to check for infection or request a faecal sample if he suspects threadworms. He may prescribe a soothing cream for the soreness.

Irritating thick white discharge from vagina
A fungal infection, thrush, is a possibility, especially if the child has been taking antibiotics or is diabetic.

Treatment: Consult your doctor. He may be able to make a diagnosis from examination, or may need to send a sample of discharge for analysis. If thrush is confirmed, anti-fungal cream or pessaries will be prescribed.

Thin white discharge
If your daughter is nearing puberty, increased hormonal discharge is quite normal. As long as there is no irritation, and the discharge is not smelly or offensive, no treatment is needed.

Greyish-yellow/greenish vaginal discharge
Can be caused by infection. Small children sometimes push foreign bodies into the vagina which lodge there and start problems.

Offensive vaginal discharge can also be a sign of sexually transmitted disease (see Women's symptoms, sexually transmitted diseases, p. 179).

Treatment: Depends on the cause of the problem.

HAIR AND SCALP PROBLEMS

Itchy scalp

Head lice is a possibility. Check behind your child's ears and at
the nape of the neck for signs of lice. They are tiny brown insects
a little larger than a grain of sugar. You may also spot 'nits', the
hatched eggs of the head lice. These look like flakes of dandruff
and stick to the hair-shaft.

Treatment: Consult your pharmacist for a suitable lotion or
shampoo for your child and follow the instructions carefully.

Examine the heads of other family members and treat them
also if infected. Buy a fine-toothed 'nit' comb and use it daily. It
removes the eggs of the head lice and prevents re-infestation.

Itchy and/or flaky scalp

The most likely cause of itching or flaking scalp is dandruff.

Treatment: Self-help measures such as regular use of a good
anti-dandruff shampoo are normally effective. If the problem persists, consult your doctor.

Bald patches

Young babies frequently develop bald patches when fine baby
hair is rubbed away by continual contact with bedclothes or the
baby-seat. The patches will disappear as new hair grows. In older
children, bald, scaly patches may be caused by a fungal infection
such as ringworm.

Treatment: Consult your doctor for older children. For ringworm, an anti-fungal ointment is often prescribed. The hair will
grow back normally once the infection has cleared. Regular washing of brushes and combs will prevent re-infection.

HEADACHE

Headache is very common in children. It may be brought on by tiredness, hunger, the onset of a cold, over-excitement, or anxiety. Keeping the child resting in a quiet room, giving a drink and a biscuit plus a dose of children's paracetamol syrup, can all help relieve the pain.

Occasional headaches are no cause for concern, but frequent headache should always be brought to your doctor's attention.

Severe headache with vomiting, high temperature, drowsiness or stiff neck can be signs of meningitis, which is a dangerous illness requiring immediate medical attention (see below).

Headache with high temperature

Infections and inflammation which cause fever can often bring on a headache (see High temperature, p. 212).

Vomiting followed by headache

Vomiting can sometimes cause headache (see Vomiting, p. 269).

Headache with vomiting and/or visual disturbance

Migraine sometimes affects older children, although it's not common. It can run in families. A migraine headache may be preceded by sickness and stomachache. The child may look pale and complain of seeing flashing lights. The headache may affect one side of the head only. The cause of migraine in children and adults is unknown. Children sometimes grow out of the condition.

Certain foods, such as cheese or chocolate, tend to trigger attacks in some sufferers.

Treatment: Follow the measures described above to help relieve pain. Give children's paracetamol as soon as possible to help avoid a severe attack. If your child suffers regularly, try to pinpoint any foods that tend to trigger an attack. Severe or frequent headaches need to be referred to your doctor. Strong anti-migraine drugs are available, but doctors tend to avoid prescribing these for children if possible.

Headaches after reading or other close work

Such headaches may be caused by visual problems such as short-sightedness. Far more commonly, they are caused by poor posture.

Treatment: See your doctor in the first instance. He may carry out a simple eye test and advise if the child should see an optician for a full check. Glasses may be necessary.

Headache with high temperature and/or drowsiness/stiff neck/vomiting without diarrhoea

These are all symptoms of meningitis, an inflammation of the membranes surrounding the brain, caused by a bacterial or viral infection. This can be a very serious illness. It needs immediate treatment. Get medical help at once from your doctor, or take the child to hospital.

Treatment: If meningitis is suspected, a lumbar puncture (see Medical diagnostic tests, p. 306) and possibly a blood test will be undertaken to confirm the diagnosis. There are two types of meningitis.

Bacterial meningitis, which is the more serious, is treated with large doses of antibiotics given by injection or drip. The child may need nursing in intensive care if the illness is severe.

Viral meningitis is a milder illness and there is no specific treatment for it.

HIGH TEMPERATURE

The mechanism that lowers body temperature is immature in babies and children under five. Because of this, they can develop a very high temperature alarmingly quickly in response to infection by bacteria or viruses. Normal body temperature can range from 36° to 37° C (97° to 99° F), and small variations are no cause for concern.

However, if a child's temperature goes above 38° C (100.4° F), he has a fever, and you should take steps to lower his temperature (see Babies under one, high temperature, p. 212). High temperature in babies and children can trigger febrile convulsions (see Fits, p. 239). If a child's temperature reaches 39° C (102° F), it is wise to call a doctor for personal advice.

The easiest way to check a child's temperature is by holding a thermometer under the arm for three minutes. In older children, put the thermometer in the mouth instead. Temperature indicator strips, which are placed on the forehead, are an alternative, possibly easier way of checking temperature, especially with babies.

High temperature with cough

Viral infections such as flu often cause a high temperature and cough.

Treatment: Take steps to lower the child's temperature if it is above 39° C (102° F) (see Babies under one, high temperature, p. 212). Make sure that he drinks plenty of fluids. Call the doctor if there's no improvement within forty-eight hours or if noisy or difficult breathing develops, or if you are worried.

High temperature with cough and fast breathing

A chest infection is possible. Call your doctor.

Treatment: The doctor will probably prescribe antibiotics. He may recommend hospital admission for a severe infection. At home, paracetamol syrup will bring down the temperature and help discomfort. Make sure that the child drinks plenty of fluids.

Inhaling may help to ease the chest.

High temperature with noisy cough and/or hoarse voice/noisy breathing

An infection of the larynx (voice box) and/or airways, sometimes called croup, is likely. However, there is also the possibility of a rare but very serious infection, epiglottitis (see below). Get medical help immediately if your child's breathing becomes difficult or loud enough to hear from a few feet away, or if he has trouble swallowing. First, it's worth trying this. Boil a kettle in the child's room for two minutes then leave the lid off, or take him into the bathroom and run two inches of very hot water into the bath. His breathing, merely by being in the room, should ease in a matter of minutes.

Treatment: A high temperature with cough may be treated at home with warm drinks and paracetamol syrup. Any breathing difficulty should be referred to your doctor. He may prescribe antibiotics or, if there is any suspicion of early epiglottitis, the child may be admitted to hospital for observation and treatment.

High temperature with loud, noisy breathing/ difficulty breathing/inability to swallow/dribbling

These are symptoms of a rare but very serious infection, epiglottitis. This is a sudden swelling of the flap at the back of the throat, the epiglottis, that closes the airways when swallowing.

If untreated, the swelling blocks breathing and can be fatal, but it is very rare.

The child will not be able to swallow and will dribble saliva because he cannot swallow it. Breathing becomes difficult and increasingly noisy. Epiglottitis develops rapidly in a matter of hours. This is a medical emergency. Get the child to hospital as quickly as possible.

The new HIB injection, given in the first year as a matter of routine, will prevent many if not all such attacks in the future. They are often caused by the *H*aemophilus *I*nfluenzae type *B* bacteria.

Treatment: The child will be given antibiotics, probably by drip, to cure the infection. He may be given oxygen or put on a ventilator to help his breathing. If the airways are obstructed, a tube may need to be inserted into the windpipe through his mouth or nose. Most children recover well within a week if treated promptly.

High temperature with sore throat

Infections of the throat and tonsils can cause sore throat and fever.

Treatment: Give children's paracetamol syrup for the temperature and pain.

Make sure that the child drinks plenty of fluids. Consult your doctor if there's no improvement within forty-eight hours. Call him at once if the child's breathing becomes noisy or difficult.

High temperature with earache or tugging at the ear in small children

A middle ear infection is a possibility, especially if the child has recently had a cold.

Treatment: Consult your doctor. He will probably prescribe a course of antibiotics. Children's paracetamol syrup given in the correct dosage can relieve pain and reduce inflammation.

High temperature with cough/runny nose/sore eyes

Measles may start with a cough, runny nose, high temperature and sore eyes (see Common childhood infectious illnesses, p. 276).

High temperature with swollen face between ear and jaw

Mumps is a possibility, especially if your child has been in contact with it during the last three weeks (see Common childhood infectious illnesses, p. 277).

High temperature with diarrhoea

Gastroenteritis, an infection of the digestive tract, is a possibility, especially if your child is also vomiting (see Diarrhoea, p. 233).

High temperature with pain on passing urine or urinating more often than normal

An infection of the urinary tract is possible.

Treatment: Consult your doctor. He will probably ask for a urine specimen. If this shows that infection is present, he will prescribe antibiotics.

High temperature with headache/vomiting without diarrhoea/drowsiness/stiff neck

These can all be symptoms of meningitis (see Headache, p. 246). This is a serious illness. Get medical help at once from your doctor, or take the child to hospital.

INJURED ARM OR LEG

Children's bumps and falls are usually harmless. From time to time, however, there is the possibility that an injury could cause a broken bone (fracture) or dislocated joint.

Pain and swelling in arm or leg following injury/limb looks misshapen/child unable to move affected limb

A broken bone or dislocated joint is possible. You should call an ambulance or get the child to hospital as quickly as you can. See Essential first aid, p. 281 for what to do while waiting for medical help.

Treatment: The limb will be examined and X-rayed at hospital if a fracture or dislocation is suspected. Fractures are usually treated by an operation to reposition the bone and 'setting' in a plaster cast or splint while the bone heals. Physiotherapy after the cast is removed helps to restore the limb to normal working.

If there is dislocation, where the arm or, more rarely, leg has been wrenched out of its socket, an operation under general anaesthetic to put it back in place is often necessary. Following this, the arm or leg may need to be rested and a further operation to stabilize the joint may subsequently be necessary.

Pain, swelling and bruising in arm or leg following injury/child can move affected limb

A sprained joint is possible. This occurs when the joint is twisted or wrenched so that some of the supporting ligaments are damaged.

Treatment: Strains and sprains can usually be treated at home following the RICE principle: R – rest the affected joint; I – ice cubes or an ice-pack will help reduce swelling, inflammation and pain (take care not to ice-burn the skin; wrap ice in a wet tea-towel before applying); C – compression (firm, but not tight, bandaging of the joint will give support and stop bleeding); E – elevation (keep an affected ankle or knee raised while resting for the next few days).

OVERWEIGHT

The problem of excess weight often begins in childhood.

Overweight children frequently grow into overweight adults who are more likely to suffer from heart and circulation problems, diabetes, and other disorders. Fat children tend to suffer from being teased; they may find it difficult to be as active as their friends; they may suffer more chest infections or tooth decay than their slimmer peers.

For these reasons, it's a good idea to keep a check on your child's weight and to take measures to reduce it if he is becoming fat. The best way to do this is to take a regular note of his weight and height and plot them on the development charts on p. 319.

If the weight-gain curve is rising more steeply than the height curve, your child is probably getting fat.

Children, like adults, gain weight when they over-eat. The vast majority of overweight people simply consume more calories than they need. Being overweight tends to run in families, usually because the whole family eat too much, or too much of the wrong things. Unhealthy eating habits established in childhood tend to persist into adult life. If you're worried about your child's weight, it could be that the whole family needs to look at its eating habits and adopt a healthier diet (see Help yourself to better health, p. 325).

Young children should never be put on a diet to make them lose weight. The aim should be to keep their weight steady while their height catches up. Seek your doctor or health visitor's advice about your child's weight and diet if you are concerned and need help. This is especially important if the child is under four.

How to help your child lose weight

- Aim for the whole family to eat a healthy diet. Eat plenty of fresh fruit and vegetables; cut down on fried foods, cakes, sausages, pies, biscuits, sweets and chocolate
- Try to stop your child eating between meals. Crisps, cake, sweets and biscuits are very high in calories. See if you can substitute fruit, bread or plain biscuits instead
- Check your child's fluid consumption. Is he drinking too much milk or too many fizzy, sugary drinks? Substitute unsweetened fruit juice or water
- Encourage your child to take more exercise. Persuade him to walk instead of riding in the pushchair. Play active outdoor games with him. Go swimming or cycling with an older child

SLEEP PROBLEMS

By the age of one, most babies regularly sleep through the night and stop waking because they are hungry. Sleep problems from then until school age are usually either due to reluctance to go to bed at all, or to unwillingness to settle down to sleep alone.

These problems are very common indeed among toddlers and pre-school children. Research has shown that at least 50 per cent of toddlers make a big fuss about going to bed at night. This, together with waking at night, can be extremely wearing for the whole family and cause a great deal of unhappiness, stress and sheer exhaustion for parents, particularly if it continues over a long period of time.

For these reasons, it is extremely worthwhile to put quite a lot of effort early on into trying to help your child become a 'good' sleeper. Establishing a bedtime routine may take time and trouble in the early days, but this is amply rewarded later on when you can be reasonably sure of evenings, and nights, to yourself without interruption.

Small babies aren't able to keep themselves awake deliberately. When they are tired they have to sleep, provided that they are not hungry or in pain. From about the age of nine months, unfortunately, babies are able to stop themselves dropping off, even when they are very tired. They may need to be coaxed and soothed to sleep.

Children all vary in the amount of sleep they need. Between nine and twelve hours is normal. A child who doesn't get as much sleep as you think he should won't physically do himself any harm. He won't stop growing or become ill. Bedtime can sometimes be more for parents' convenience than for the child's benefit. A compromise must be struck between a time that suits the child and one that gives his parents some time to themselves in the evening.

Among older children, emotional upset or anxiety, nightmares, and sometimes physical illness, can cause a child to wake in the night or prevent him sleeping.

Avoiding bedtime trouble

- Try to make bedtime as relaxed, pleasant and unhurried as possible. Avoid arguments and rows around this time. It can easily take from 5.30 to 7.30 to give a small child tea and settle him to bed, but it's time well spent if it means that you have the rest of the evening to yourself

- Establish a pleasant bedtime routine at the same time each day, and try to stick to it. A pattern such as tea, bath, television, bed, story, milk, song, or something similar, is a good one. Children are creatures of habit and find routine reassuring

- Make the child's bedroom a pleasant place with his own toys and an attractive cot or bed. Try not to use the threat of being put to bed as a punishment during the day
- Many small children are afraid of being left alone at night and will want you with them until they fall asleep. Fear of being left alone can make them reluctant to go to bed. Fifteen or twenty minutes spent sitting with a child until he drops off can be time well spent. It's better than an hour of crying and frustration
- Beware of trying to put a child who really isn't tired to bed because it's 'bedtime'. It can mean an hour of crying and irritation on both sides, time which might have been better spent looking at books or playing a quiet game together
- If a child is still sleeping two or three hours during the day, it may mean that he's not tired at bedtime. Try cutting down on daytime sleeps

Regular waking in the night

Most children, and many adults too, wake one or more times during the night. The difference between children who are 'good' and those who are 'bad' sleepers is that the 'good' sleepers can go back to sleep again on their own, whereas 'bad' sleepers will call for their parents and may cry and make a big fuss about returning to sleep.

'Bad' sleepers may simply have got into the habit of getting your attention if they wake at night. Try to keep contact during the night to a minimum. If the child wakes and doesn't drift off again after a few minutes, go to him to check that all is well, offer a drink if this is wanted, but not a nice cosy breastfeed or bottle of milk, and then leave quickly. If he cries, leave him for five minutes, reassure again briefly, and then leave. Each time he cries, lengthen the interval between your return visits, and keep your contact brief. The idea is to put across the message that you are not available for unlimited time during the night, and that long and loud crying doesn't secure any extra attention.

Waking crying in the night

Pain or discomfort may make small children who are normally good sleepers wake in the night. High temperature and coughs and colds with a runny nose may also cause children to wake because they have trouble breathing (see High temperature, p. 248, and Colds, p. 227).

In this case, a soothing drink or some children's paracetamol syrup to reduce pain and inflammation may be helpful. The child should be checked by your doctor to treat the cause of the pain if necessary.

Waking frightened in the night

Many small children wake in the night because of bad dreams or nightmares. This is common, and nothing to be alarmed about. Go to the child quickly. A good cuddle and possibly a drink is all that's usually needed.

Older children may find periods of change or disruption stressful enough to disturb their sleep. A new school, parental separation or divorce, can cause anxiety that disrupts sleep. Give comfort when he wakes in the night and try to discuss the problem with him.

SLOW GROWTH

Most parents worry from time to time, usually unnecessarily, about their children's growth. Fortunately, serious disorders causing growth problems are extremely rare. Temporary factors such as illness or anxiety, leading to loss of appetite, can sometimes interrupt the child's normal growth pattern, but this is quickly recovered once the child is well again.

Children tend naturally to go through phases of rapid and then slower growth. A baby gains weight very rapidly until the age of six months, at which time growth slows down. Around puberty, there is again a very rapid increase in weight and height. Keeping a regular check on your child's height and weight (see Children's development charts, p. 319) is the best way to avoid unnecessary anxiety.

Treatment: If you are concerned about your child's slow growth, your should see your doctor. If he confirms that your child is not growing at the expected rate, he may arrange for specialist assessment. Blood tests to check on growth hormone can be undertaken, and appropriate treatment given if this is found to be deficient.

SORE THROAT

Sore throats are very common in children. They often accompany colds and coughs. Although they are generally caused by a bacterial infection, and should give no cause for concern, they are nevertheless very painful and distressing for the child.

Tonsillitis, infection of the tonsils, and pharyngitis, infection of the throat usually caused by a cold, are the most common causes of sore throats. Occasionally, a sore throat can be an early symptom of mumps (see Common childhood infectious illnesses, p. 275).

If your child has a sore throat you can help him by:

- giving plenty of cold drinks
- giving children's paracetamol syrup to relieve the pain
- giving an older child the local chemist's recommended gargle

SPEECH DISORDERS

Many parents worry because their child seems to them late in learning to speak, speaks unclearly, or stammers. Usually, there is no cause for concern, and these problems right themselves perfectly well in time. If, however, there is a serious problem, the help of a trained speech therapist can do a great deal to improve matters.

Slow language development

Every child develops at his own pace, but generally, by the age of two, most children will have a vocabulary of at least 100 words, and will be starting to put two-word sentences together, for example 'Mummy come' or 'Want juice'. Slow development, where the child is slow to understand speech or is able to use very few words, can be caused by a number of factors. Deafness is the most common one (see Deafness, p. 232), but lack of stimulation and parental conversation, emotional disturbance or, in a few cases, limited intelligence, can also have an effect.

There are a few groups of children in which slow language development is fairly common and is no cause for concern:

- Boys tend to be later talkers than girls
- Twins may be slower to speak. They may receive less parental attention than a single child, and often communicate with each other non-verbally without the need for speech, or by using a 'private' language
- Younger children in a large family may get less attention; older brothers or sisters may speak for them or interpret their wishes without the need for words

Treatment: Most children who are late or slow in talking catch up with their peers very quickly once they start. However, if your doctor suspects a problem he may give the child a hearing test, or refer him to a specialist. If there is a problem, specialist speech therapy or language-based learning assistance from a specialist teacher can help.

Stammering

This is common in children between the ages of two and four. It's usually just part of the child's natural difficulty in finding the right words. Stammering generally dies out naturally, but about half of all children who still stammer at the age of five will carry on into adulthood. Anxiety about the condition makes it worse.

Treatment: Help from a speech therapist, if given in the early years, will usually overcome the difficulty.

Lisping, poor articulation

Many small children have difficulty pronouncing certain sounds or combinations of sounds while they are learning to speak. Usually this will sort itself out in time. Continually correcting the child only makes him miserable or self-conscious. If the problem is so bad that it stops others understanding him by the time he is school age, see your doctor.

Treatment: Very occasionally, a structural abnormality of the mouth, lips, tongue, palate, throat or larynx can hinder normal speech. Your doctor will examine your child and, if necessary, send him to a specialist, who will investigate further and take appropriate action.

SPOTS AND RASHES

Children frequently develop spots and rashes that disappear as quickly as they come. Usually these are nothing to worry about.

However, spots or rashes that cause high temperature, sickness, or make the child feel generally unwell, should be reported to your doctor. They can be signs of an infectious illness (see Common childhood infectious illnesses, p. 275). Even children who have been vaccinated may sometimes catch these illnesses, so don't discount them even if your child has been 'jabbed'.

Spots and rashes can also be caused by an allergic reaction to irritants such as chemicals. An itchy or sore rash that doesn't clear up with ordinary soothing-creams in a few days should be reported to your doctor.

Spots or rash with high temperature

This usually means that the child has caught one of the common infectious illnesses (see Common childhood infectious illnesses, p. 275).

Measles, chickenpox, or roseola infantum are possibilities. These illnesses may sometimes give an older child more trouble than a younger one. They should always be seen by a doctor in a baby less than one year, and in older children if you are worried.

Itchy, red, scaly, weeping or blistery rash

Childhood (atopic) eczema is likely. Eczema is an allergic reaction. Children who get hay fever and/or asthma often suffer with eczema too. It tends to run in families.

Childhood eczema can start in babyhood with bad nappy rash.

It frequently then goes on to affect the hands and wrists, the creases of the arms, and behind the knees. In bad cases, the face and trunk can also be involved. Eczema can be intensely itchy and upsetting for the child.

Treatment: Mild cases can be treated at home. Avoid irritating the skin with soap. Emulsifying ointment, which can be bought at the chemist's, should be used instead to clean and moisturize.

Additional unscented emollient creams can also help counteract dryness and itching. Avoid woollens next to the skin. Cotton clothes are softer and let the skin breathe.

If the rash is weepy or very widespread, consult your doctor.

He may prescribe a strong steroid cream which can clear the skin but should be used as sparingly as possible. Prolonged or excessive use can cause thinning of the skin and lead to an increased risk of infection. If the skin is infected, antibiotics may be prescribed. Anti-histamines as syrup or tablets to stop the itching can help if the rash is causing sleeplessness, especially in younger children.

Red, scaly, weepy rash that dries with golden yellow crusts

Impetigo is a possibility. This is a bacterial skin infection which is highly contagious and seems to affect children more than adults.

Treatment: Consult your doctor. He will prescribe an antibiotic cream. Carefully wash the crusts away with warm water. It's important not to share towels or flannels while the infection persists, to guard against other family members getting it.

Patches of bright-red, raised spots, very itchy

Urticaria, nettle rash or hives, is an allergic skin reaction. It can be caused by foods, drugs, chemicals or plants.

Treatment: Normally the rash subsides leaving no trace within about four hours. Calamine lotion can soothe the itching in the meantime. Your chemist may suggest an antihistamine medicine.

Occasionally, in severe cases, there is wheezing or swelling of the mouth or face. This can be dangerous, and you should get medical help at once.

Patches of red, flaky skin, sore or itchy

Dermatitis, a term which simply means inflamed skin, can be caused by coming into contact with substances that cause irritation. It can be caused by perfumed soaps or toiletries in children with sensitive skin. Babies' nappy rash is a form of dermatitis.

Treatment: Try to discover the cause of the inflammation and avoid it. Use emulsifying ointment, available from the chemist's, to cleanse and moisturize the skin. Mild hydrocortisone creams are now available from the chemist's without prescription. These quickly relieve itching and inflammation.

Circle of itchy, red, scaly skin with a bumpy edge

This is probably ringworm, a fungal infection which is contagious. It can be caught from animals. If it affects the scalp, it can cause bald patches.

Treatment: Your doctor will prescribe an anti-fungal cream or lotion, and possibly a drug to be taken orally if the infection is widespread.

The cream or lotion will need to be used for a few weeks after the infection has cleared up to prevent it recurring.

Wash all the child's brushes and combs, towels and face-flannels, and keep them separate from everyone else's. Stop him scratching infected spots if at all possible. Make sure that he washes his hands after touching them, so as not to spread the infection to other places.

One or several raised red spots, very itchy and inflamed

Flea or mosquito or other insect bites are a possibility.

Treatment: Calamine lotion on the affected area can be very soothing. If the inflammation is severe, mild anti-histamine creams can be bought at the chemist's without prescription. Try to stop the child scratching and so infecting the spots.

Itchy raised red or grey lines between fingers, at wrists or elbows

Scabies, an infection from a small parasite, is possible.

Treatment: See your doctor. He will prescribe a lotion containing insecticide. This must be applied all over, and the entire family must be treated at the same time to avoid re-infection. The treatment needs to be repeated again after twenty-four hours. Bedding, towels and clothing should all be laundered at the same time to destroy the mite.

Blackheads, whiteheads, inflamed spots, painful red lumps under the skin

These are all symptoms of acne, which many children suffer from to some degree as they approach their teens. It's caused by an excess production of the skin's natural oils due to hormonal activity.

Pores become blocked and infection and inflammation set in.

Treatment: Self-help measures such as anti-bacterial face-washes, lotions and soaps can help in mild cases, but persistence is important. Most users stop too quickly. For many, the advice will be to continue for three months, or continually, if the rash returns when it's stopped. Creams containing benzol or sulphur, which peels the top layer of the skin, can help, but use carefully as they can cause soreness.

If the acne doesn't clear, see your doctor. Antibiotics and other preparations can help greatly and prevent permanent scarring.

SWOLLEN GLANDS

Children are very prone to swollen glands as a result of infection. Those near the surface of the skin, on either side of the neck, under the arms, and in the groin, are most noticeable, but in fact there are lymph glands throughout the body. Usually, swollen glands are no cause for concern, although they may feel rather tender. However, very painful or persistently swollen glands should be seen by your doctor.

Swelling under the chin and behind the ear with high temperature, headache, loss of appetite

These are all symptoms of mumps (see Common childhood infectious illnesses, p. 277).

Swelling at the back of the neck and behind the ears and slight temperature/runny nose/feeling unwell

German measles causes the lymph glands at the back of the neck and behind the ears to swell (see Common childhood infectious illnesses, p. 275).

Swelling under the chin and behind the ear and/or under the arms, in the groin with fever/headache/ feeling generally unwell/sore throat

Glandular fever (infectious mononucleosis), a viral illness, is a possibility.

Treatment; There is no specific treatment for glandular fever.

Children's paracetamol syrup can relieve fever and discomfort, and plenty of fluids are advised. Unfortunately, feeling unwell and tired may continue for many weeks or even months. A doctor may take a blood test to confirm glandular fever if such symptoms persist.

Swelling down the sides of the neck and sore throat

Tonsillitis often causes swelling of the lymph glands near the tonsils. The child may also have a slight temperature and be unwilling to eat because of a painful throat.

Treatment: Children's paracetamol syrup can relieve the pain. Give the child plenty of cold drinks, but don't force food on him if he doesn't want to eat. If the sore throat persists for more than two days, see your doctor. He may prescribe antibiotics if appropriate. An operation to remove the tonsils is now rarely performed, only in cases of severe recurring infection.

TOOTHACHE

Toothache is caused when bacteria in the mouth act on sugar and produce acids which attack tooth enamel. There are some very simple steps you can take to ensure that your child never suffers the misery of toothache. They are:

- Make sure that your child's teeth are cleaned daily from the moment they arrive. Clean a tiny baby's teeth yourself with a smear of toothpaste on a soft cloth. Teach a toddler to handle a toothbrush and explain why it's important to clean teeth. Allow him to 'clean' himself, and follow his attempts with a thorough cleaning yourself. Make sure that you check that older children are cleaning thoroughly by using disclosing tablets that show up missed plaque from time to time
- Sugar is the main cause of dental decay. Restrict the amount of sweets and sweet drinks your child consumes. Try to make sure that sweets are eaten quickly and aren't the type that are sucked for several hours. Never give children sweet drinks for

the night after they've cleaned their teeth, only plain water.
Never put sweet juices on a baby's dummy. Sugar will be in
contact with his teeth all day and can inflict real damage
• Visit your dentist regularly
• Fluoride drops or tablets can help prevent tooth decay. They
  are only necessary in areas where fluoride is not already added
  to, or present in the water. Check with your dentist, doctor or
  health visitor before giving extra fluoride. Overdosing can give
  children mottled-looking teeth

Pain on eating and drinking/sensitivity to hot and cold foods

It's likely that your child has tooth decay. See the dentist at once.
  Treatment: Your dentist will take appropriate action, probably
a filling or extraction, and explain how to prevent this happening
again.

Pain after visiting the dentist

If your child has a new filling, there is often some pain when
biting on it at first. This should subside after a few days. If not,
go back to the dentist. A filling that's too 'high' can cause discomfort when eating. Your dentist will adjust the filling if
necessary.

UNUSUAL BREATHING

Breathing abnormally in a baby or child should always be taken
seriously. Abnormal breathing includes difficulty in breathing or
breathlessness, loud, noisy breathing, wheezing or grunting, and
very fast breathing (more than fifty breaths a minute is never

normal except after exercise). If your child exhibits noisy breathing plus any of the following symptoms:

- blueness of the tongue or lips
- drowsiness
- fast breathing
- difficulty speaking or making sounds

it is a medical emergency and you should get him to hospital at once.

Noisy, fast breathing

A chest infection, especially if the child has recently had a cold and has developed a cough, is possible.

Treatment: See your doctor. In severe cases the child is likely to be admitted to hospital. If he is being treated at home, the doctor is likely to prescribe antibiotics and recommend plenty of fluids and keeping the child warm in bed.

Sudden difficulty breathing with wheezing, noisy breathing and/or any of the symptoms listed above

A severe asthma attack is possible. This is a medical emergency and you should get the child to hospital immediately. Asthma is an allergic reaction often provoked by dust, house mites, pollen and other irritants. However, in some children a first asthma attack can be brought on by a cold or other viral infection.

Never under-estimate the severity of asthma attacks.

Treatment: Oxygen and drugs to ease breathing will be given, and the child will probably be admitted to hospital. He will be assessed to determine whether he should regularly take medicines to prevent further attacks.

Sudden noisy breathing with any of the symptoms listed above, children under four years

Croup, an infection and inflammation of the throat and windpipe causing swelling, is a medical emergency in young children. If the child also has a high temperature and dribbles, these are symptoms of a rare but very serious infection, epiglottitis (see High temperature, p. 248). This is a sudden swelling of the flap at the back of the throat, the epiglottis, that closes the airways when swallowing. If untreated the swelling blocks breathing and can be fatal – but it is rare.

Treatment: Get the child to hospital immediately. The child will be given oxygen to help breathing, or be put on a ventilator in serious cases, and be given antibiotics and fluids by drip.

URINARY PROBLEMS

If your child experiences pain on passing urine, or if he begins to urinate much more frequently than normal, he should see a doctor.

Stinging or pain on passing urine/urinating much more often than normal/high temperature

An infection of the urinary tract is likely. This is much more common in girls than in boys. It is easier for bacteria from the bowel to reach the urinary tract and set up an infection in girls.

Treatment: The doctor will ask for a urine specimen to confirm an infection. A course of antibiotics will usually be prescribed if infection is found.

Passing large volumes of urine/urinating often with weight loss and/or tiredness/very thirsty

Diabetes can cause these symptoms. If the pancreas fails to produce enough insulin, the body isn't able to convert the sugars in food into energy. As a result, the child loses weight, feels tired all the time, and glucose is excreted in the urine.

Treatment: Consult your doctor. A simple test will show the presence of glucose in the urine. If diabetes is confirmed, the child will be referred to a specialist. Insulin will need to be taken, usually by injection, to provide what the body cannot make, and adjustments made to diet.

VISUAL DISORDERS

Problems with eyesight are relatively common in children.

Fortunately, most are picked up by regular eye tests at clinics and schools. However, if you suspect that your child has a problem with his sight that's been overlooked, see a doctor at once. He will arrange a full eye test. Visual problems, if not corrected, can cause learning difficulties.

VOMITING

Vomiting in children can be caused by something as trivial as over-excitement or eating too much of the wrong foods. It can sometimes herald the start of a cold or other type of infection.

It can be caused by stress or car sickness. Often there's no apparent reason for an occasional bout of sickness.

Sometimes, however, vomiting can be a sign of serious illness if accompanied by certain danger signs. You should call the doctor directly if a child:

- experiences continuous abdominal pain for more than three hours
- has frequent bouts of vomiting for more than twelve hours
- refuses to drink
- has sunken eyes
- has a dry tongue
- is more than usually drowsy
- passes no urine for over six hours
- vomits greenish-yellow matter
- experiences vomiting with fever/headache/stiff neck/unusual drowsiness

Vomiting with abdominal pain for over three hours

Appendicitis is a possibility.

Treatment: Appendicitis is a medical emergency. Get the child to hospital as quickly as possible. Don't give anything to eat or drink since surgery may be necessary to investigate the cause of the pain and remove the appendix if it is found to be inflamed.

An operation to remove the appendix is straightforward. The child will be in hospital for up to a week and most children recover quickly afterwards.

Vomiting with diarrhoea

Gastroenteritis, an inflammation of the digestive tract, is likely (see Diarrhoea, p. 233).

Vomiting greenish-yellow matter with diarrhoea

Gastroenteritis is most likely. However, there are other possibilities. Give the child only plain water to drink. If pain is persistent, and continues for over three hours, treat as for appendicitis.

Vomiting with high temperature, frequent urination or bedwetting

A urinary tract infection is possible (see Urinary problems, p. 268).

Vomiting after violent bouts of coughing

Whooping cough causes vomiting after coughing fits. You should see your doctor at once.

Vomiting with high temperature/unusual drowsiness and/or headache/stiff neck

Meningitis, an inflammation of the membrane surrounding the brain, can cause such symptoms (see Headache, p. 246). This is a serious illness and needs immediate medical help. See your doctor at once, or take the child straight to hospital.

COMMON CHILDHOOD INFECTIOUS ILLNESSES

COMMON CHILDHOOD INFECTIOUS ILLNESSES

CHICKENPOX

A very infectious viral disease spread by droplet infection and by direct contact. It tends to be a mild illness in children but more serious in adults. The incubation period (the time between first contact with the disease and the development of symptoms) is twelve to twenty-one days. The child is infectious from five days before the rash appears until all the spots have dry scabs.

Symptoms: Mild fever, headache, and general feeling of being unwell. Raised red spots rapidly turning to itchy blisters on trunk, face and, sometimes, scalp. The spots gradually dry to forms crusts that can last for a few weeks.

Treatment: Fever can be treated with children's paracetamol syrup. Calamine lotion is useful for soothing itchy spots. Keep your child's nails short and try to discourage scratching, which can cause infection and scarring.

GERMAN MEASLES (RUBELLA)

A viral infection spread by droplets.

This is a mild illness in children, but can be more troublesome in adults. It is very serious if contracted by a woman in the early months of pregnancy; it can cause birth defects in the unborn child. The incubation period is fourteen to twenty-one days. A child can pass on the infection a week before his own symptoms show, and is infectious for up to five days after the rash has gone.

Symptoms: A rash of fine pink spots over the face and trunk, which gradually merge. There may be a slight fever, swollen glands in the neck and/or a runny nose. Some children have such mild symptoms that the illness goes unnoticed.

Treatment: There is no specific treatment. Children's paracetamol syrup may be given for raised temperature. Care should be taken to avoid contact with any women who are pregnant. Recovery normally takes up to ten days, but usually much less.

MEASLES

A viral infection spread by droplets sneezed or coughed from the mouth and nose. Measles is highly infectious from just before the first symptoms begin until about four days after the rash appears. The incubation period is seven to fourteen days.

Symptoms: First, a very runny nose with red eyes and a dry cough, followed by fever. About four days later, a rash of dull red spots, which soon merge into blotches, appears. They show first behind the ears, and rapidly spread to the face and trunk. The rash fades over a few days, and the skin becomes dry and scaly.

Treatment: If you suspect measles, telephone your doctor for advice. Don't take the child to the doctor's surgery; he may infect others. It is not necessary for the child to go to bed unless he wants to. Give children's paracetamol syrup for high temperature if needed. Recovery normally takes about ten days.

MUMPS

A viral infection spread by droplets. Can be more serious in adults, especially male, than in children. The child is infectious for a week before he develops symptoms and for a week after.

The incubation period is twelve to twenty-one days.

Symptoms: Fever, feeling generally unwell, headache and loss of appetite. Sore throat and swollen glands in the neck, below, in front of, and behind the ears.

Treatment: Pain and fever can be treated with paracetamol syrup. The child may need to have a liquid diet, since the sore throat can make it painful to eat. Recovery takes about ten days.

ROSEOLA INFANTUM

A fairly common infection affecting children between six months and two years. The incubation period varies but is around ten days. The child is infectious for five days after symptoms have appeared.

Symptoms: Sudden high fever followed by fine pink rash that spreads rapidly over the body. Once the rash appears, the temperature returns to normal.

Treatment: Give children's paracetamol syrup for high temperature if necessary.

ESSENTIAL FIRST AID

ESSENTIAL FIRST AID

Prompt and correct first aid to victims of serious accidents can save lives. Fortunately, most of us are only ever called upon to deal with life's minor emergencies. However, there is a right and a wrong way to treat even slight cuts or burns, and in serious cases being able to take the correct action quickly while waiting for medical help to arrive really is a matter of life and death.

There is no substitute for classes in first aid. Techniques such as mouth-to-mouth resuscitation are best learned by doing them for real.

Even so, becoming familiar with the right way of dealing with emergencies by reading the following instructions could help you act swiftly and correctly in an emergency.

EMERGENCY CHECKLIST

There are three emergency situations which are life-threatening:

1   lack of breathing or heartbeat
2   severe bleeding
3   unconsciousness

Certain parts of the body – vital nerve cells in the brain, for example – can die if deprived of oxygen for as little as three minutes. It's vital. therefore, that a person continues to take oxygen into his lungs after an accident, and that the oxygen circulates around the body in the blood.

The St John Ambulance organization has an ABC rule to help first-aiders remember the action they should take:

A an open airway
B adequate breathing
C sufficient circulation

MOUTH-TO-MOUTH RESUSCITATION

If a casualty is not breathing, and the heart does not appear to be beating, it's vital that you begin mouth-to-mouth resuscitation straightaway. These are the steps to take.

A Open the airway. After an accident, the airway may be closed. If the person is unconscious, his head may have lolled forward or the tongue dropped back, narrowing or blocking the airway. Saliva or vomit in the back of the throat can do the same thing
  1 Lay the victim on his back, face upward
  2 Tip the head well back by lifting the chin up with your fingers. The tongue will be lifted clear of the airway as you do this
  3 Use your first two fingers to scoop out any blockage. Once the airway is open, the casualty may begin breathing spontaneously. If not, begin resuscitation at once

B Breathing
  1 Open your mouth wide and take a deep breath. Pinch the casualty's nose and seal your mouth around his. Blow strongly into his mouth until you see his chest rise (Figures i and ii)
  2 Watch the casualty's chest fall, take a deep breath and blow again
  3 Continue to give a breath every five seconds until breathing is restored or medical help arrives

If there is no pulse or heartbeat, external cardiac massage should be started. To understand the signs and symptoms so that you know when to start and when you're making it work properly, you really need to take a course. I recommend that you do.

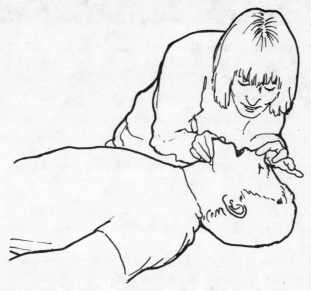

Figure (i)

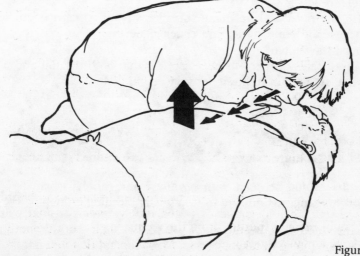

Figure (ii)

THE RECOVERY POSITION

A person who is unconscious but breathing should be placed in
this position. It allows him to breathe and prevents choking. DO
NOT use this position if the person could have a back injury.

1 Kneel beside the casualty. First check the person's mouth.
   Remove false teeth or anything the person could choke on.
   Turn the casualty's head towards you and tilt it back to keep
   the airway open (Figure iii)
2 Straighten the casualty's legs. Place the arm nearest you out
   at right angles to the body, elbow bent, and with the palm
   uppermost (Figure iv)
3 Bring the arm furthest from you across the chest and hold
   the hand, palm outwards, against the casualty's nearest cheek
   (Figure v)
4 With your other hand, grasp the thigh furthest from you and
   pull the knee up, keeping the foot flat on the ground
5 Keeping his hand pressed against his cheek, pull at the
   casualty's thigh to roll him towards you and on to his side
   (Figure vi)
6 Tilt the head back to make sure the airway remains open.
   Adjust the hand under the cheek if necessary, so that the
   head stays tilted
7 Adjust the upper leg, if necessary, so that both the hip and
   knee are bent at right-angles (Figure vii)

BLEEDING

Bleeding should be dealt with promptly and calmly. It can be
very distressing. Act quickly to stop severe bleeding if the blood:

- is bright red and spurting from the wound
- a large amount is being lost

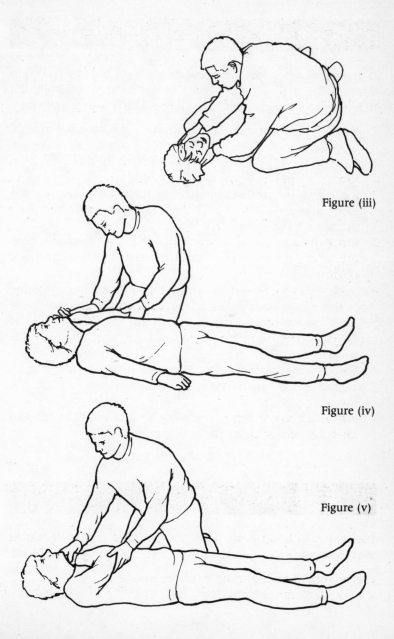

Figure (iii)

Figure (iv)

Figure (v)

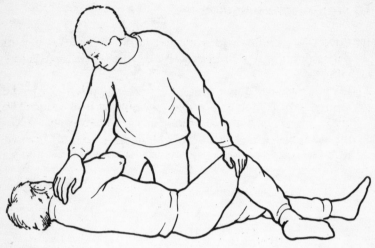

Figure (vi)

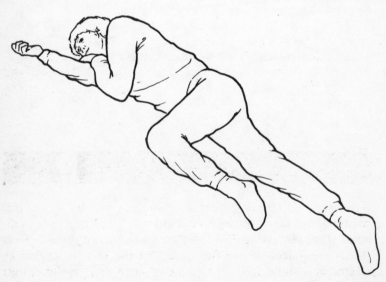

Figure (vii)

To stop severe bleeding

1 Cover the wound with a clean (sterile, if possible) pad of material, and press firmly to reduce the blood flow (Figure viii)
2 Lay the casualty down in a comfortable position. Raise the injured part as high as possible and support it to reduce the blood flow, continuing to press hard on the dressing
3 Bind the pad firmly over the wound. If it becomes soaked with blood, add another pad and bind again; don't remove it (Figure ix)

Minor cuts and grazes

1 Allow the wound to bleed freely for a few seconds. This cleans it. The bleeding will usually stop of its own accord after a short while. Pressing a clean pad over it will help to stop the bleeding
2 Once bleeding has stopped, clean around the wound carefully with clear water
3 Small cuts and grazes heal more quickly if left uncovered
4 Any cut that is longer than 1 cm (½ in), or that is dirty and deep (puncture wounds, say, from a nail), should be seen by a doctor

BURNS

Burns may be caused by dry heat such as fire, by moist heat (steam or hot liquids), corrosive chemicals, electricity, or by radiation (sunburn). Burns covering an area of more than 2–3 cm (1 in), going deeper than the surface of the skin, or caused by electricity, require medical treatment, since there is the danger of infection and of shock.

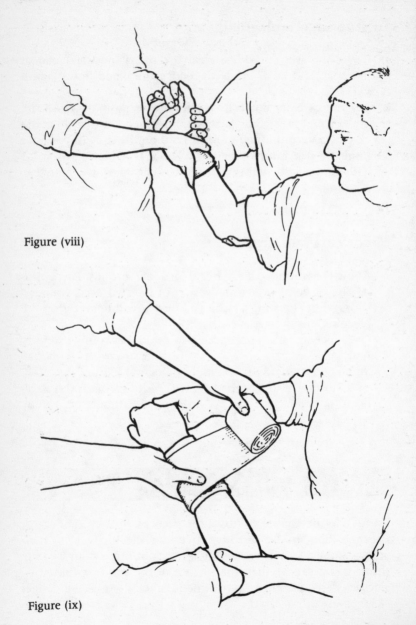

Figure (viii)

Figure (ix)

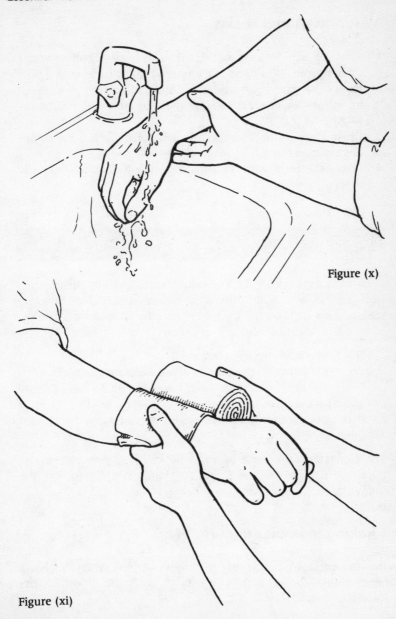

Figure (x)

Figure (xi)

Minor burns and scalds

1 Remove any clothing that's soaked in hot fat, boiling water, or chemicals. Don't remove anything that's sticking to a burn
2 Hold the injured part under running cold water, or immerse in water, for at least ten minutes, or until the pain stops (Figure x)
3 Do not apply any creams, fat or lotions. Do not break any blisters that form
4 Cover the burn with a clean, dry, non-fluffy, non-adhesive dressing (Figure xi)

CHOKING

If an adult chokes on food, and is unable to cough up the obstruction, he will need help, otherwise breathing may stop. First, try several firm slaps on the back between the shoulder-blades.

As a last resort try abdominal thrusts:

1 Hold the victim up from behind
2 Press one fist with the thumb inward against the waist
3 Grasp your fist with your other hand and give a hard inward and upward thrust under the rib-cage (Figure xii)
4 If the obstruction is not dislodged, repeat again up to four times

The same technique can be used for children over nine using only one fist and far less force. For younger children, use the following methods.

Choking in babies under a year

Be very careful when trying to remove any obstruction from a small child's throat; it is very easy to push the object further down.

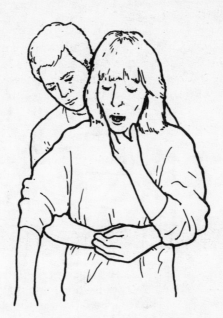

Figure (xii)

1 Lay the baby face down on your forearm along your lap with his head lower than his body. Support his chest with your hand
2 Slap him sharply between the shoulder-blades several times

Choking in children up to nine years

1 Place the child face down across your lap
2 Give several sharp blows between the shoulder-blades (Figure xiii)

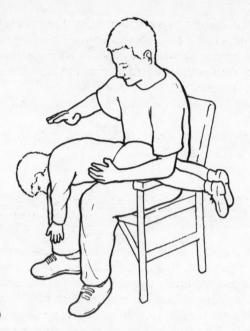

Figure (xiii)

DROWNING

If someone is drowning, check their breathing as soon as you reach them. If they are not breathing, remove any obstacles such as seaweed from the mouth, and begin mouth-to-mouth resuscitation (see above) at once if you can. Don't stop to get them out of the water or to remove water from the lungs; just aim to restore breathing as quickly as possible and then get medical help.

ELECTRIC SHOCK

Severe electric shock can knock a person unconscious, can cause the heart to stop beating, and can inflict severe burns.

1 Break the current by switching off at the mains, if possible; otherwise, push the victim away from the source of electricity using a broom or wooden chair or stool. Never touch the casualty with your bare hands unless you are certain that the current is turned off
2 If the person is unconscious, give mouth-to-mouth resuscitation
3 Once breathing has started, place in the recovery position (see above) and call help

POISONING

Accidental poisoning with household chemicals, medicines, alcohol, or poisonous plants or berries is one of the most common reasons for children under five to be admitted to hospital. Poisoning in adults is more likely to be the result of a drug overdose, either accidental or deliberate. Drowsiness or confusion, vomiting or diarrhoea, breathing difficulty or unconsciousness, can all result from poisoning.

1 Try to get some information from the casualty, or to discover yourself what has been swallowed and how much. This will help doctors give the correct treatment
2 Do not induce vomiting
3 Place the casualty in the recovery position (see above), even if he is not unconscious (he may vomit at any time) until medical help arrives

SHOCK

Shock is a serious condition which can even be fatal. It can be the result of severe injuries, large loss of blood, burns or electrocution. The casualty's blood pressure drops dramatically; he may become pale and sweaty, breathe fast or gulp air, complain of thirst, be drowsy or confused.

1 Don't move the person more than is necessary. Offer lots of reassurance
2 Treat any cause you can remedy, such as severe bleeding
3 Lay him down flat on his back. Raise his legs
4 Keep him warm with a coat or blanket (Figure xiv)
5 Do not give anything to eat or drink

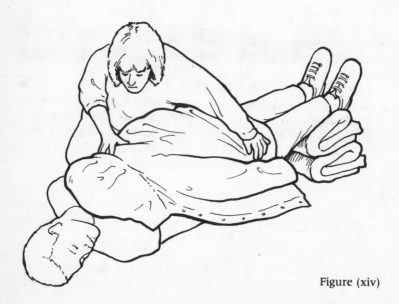

Figure (xiv)

HOME FIRST AID KIT

It is always useful to have a small first aid kit ready at home to deal with minor medical emergencies. It should be stored in a clean, air-tight container that can be locked, or that is out of reach of children.

It should include:

- a clinical thermometer
- antiseptic cream for cuts and scrapes
- insect sting reliever
- indigestion medicine or tablets
- aspirin or paracetamol
- calamine lotion
- petroleum jelly
- surgical spirit
- a packet of sterile cotton wool
- two large, two medium, two small sterile bandages with dressings
- a packet of sterile gauze dressing
- two sterile triangular bandages
- waterproof plasters
- surgical tape
- tweezers
- scissors
- safety pins

MEDICAL
DIAGNOSTIC TESTS

MEDICAL
DIAGNOSTIC TESTS

A doctor uses a number of techniques to detect and diagnose illness. Perhaps the most important is listening to and taking note of his patient's symptoms and medical history. Usually, a physical examination is performed too if this is appropriate. In addition to these time-honoured methods, there are an increasing number of specialized medical tests that can be used to help confirm or arrive at the diagnosis of a problem, or to check the progress of an illness or the effectiveness of treatment.

Medical tests which look for disease or confirm its presence take several forms. Clinical laboratory tests involve taking a sample of body fluids, or products such as urine, blood, faeces, spinal fluid, sputum, sweat or saliva, to look for evidence of infection or body chemicals which are at higher or lower levels than normal, or which should not be there.

Imaging techniques, such as X-rays, ultrasound scans, CT (computerized tomography) scanning, magnetic resonance imaging, and others, use a variety of methods to examine the body's organs and tissues and to detect any abnormalities.

Scoping techniques use a variety of viewing devices to look directly at, or inside, the body's organs and cavities. The development of fibre optics in recent years has been a major advance. Minute viewing instruments can now be inserted into the smallest body space, and can even see around corners or past obstacles. Some can take samples of tissue for analysis and carry out other procedures, at the same time avoiding the need for 'open' surgery.

These are some of the most commonly performed medical diagnostic tests.

ANGIOGRAPHY

This is a form of X-ray used to examine the arteries – called arteriography – and check if they have become narrowed or blocked. The same method is also used for veins and is called venography.

A sedative drug is usually given before a small tube is inserted into an artery in the arm or leg. The catheter is passed along the blood vessel until it reaches the area which is to be examined. A dye which shows up on X-rays is then released into the bloodstream and X-rays of the area are taken.

BARIUM X-RAY

Barium sulphate is a metallic salt that shows up on X-ray pictures. It is used to examine areas of the digestive tract. A barium meal, or barium swallow, is a drink given before X-rays of the gullet, stomach or small intestine are taken. If X-rays are needed of the large intestine, colon or rectum, a barium enema is given.

Patients are usually asked to eat nothing after midnight before either procedure. A laxative is given to clear the bowel before a barium enema.

BIOPSY

A biopsy is the removal of a small piece of body tissue for examination under the microscope. This test is often used to diagnose cancer. There are several ways of collecting a sample for biopsy. The method depends on the site of the cells that are needed. A needle biopsy uses a fine needle inserted into the organ to draw off a few cells. An endoscopic biopsy uses a viewing-tube with a small instrument attached which is inserted where required in order to remove cells. Small skin lumps are usually removed completely for biopsy. Once the cells are taken, they are sent to the laboratory for analysis.

BLADDER FUNCTION TEST

This test is performed to investigate cases of unstable bladder and incontinence. There are several parts to the test. The first requires measuring the volume of the bladder. You will be asked to drink a large quantity of liquid and then empty your bladder.

A catheter is then inserted and the bladder filled with radio-opaque liquid which will show up on X-ray. Pictures are taken while urination takes place. Other tests involve measuring the pressure inside the bladder when urinating and when at rest using pressure-sensitive probes. These tests are not particularly pleasant for the patient, but do give doctors a great deal of valuable information.

BLOOD TEST

Blood acts as the body's transport system, carrying oxygen, nutrients, waste products, hormones and proteins to the cells.

Blood tests can give doctors valuable information about the health of the body's major organs, tell him how well the lungs and heart are working, show any hormonal imbalance or metabolic disorders, or detect the presence of infection. There are three main types of blood tests. Haematological tests look at the numbers, the size, shapes and appearance of the white and red blood cells themselves. Biochemical tests measure the levels of various chemicals which are dissolved in the blood. Microbiological tests check for the presence of bacteria and viruses in the blood, and the levels of antibodies formed against them.

A sample of about 20 ml of blood is needed for most tests. It is usually taken from a vein in the arm with a sterile needle that's discarded after use. The procedure takes minutes only and is not painful. If only a few drops are needed, the blood is taken by pricking a finger or thumb. Most blood samples are sent to a laboratory for analysis. However, there are a few simple tests that GPs undertake in their own surgeries.

BRONCHOSCOPY

This is an examination of the main airways of the lungs, the bronchi, using a viewing-instrument. The fibre optic broncho-scope is a flexible thin tube which is passed into the body via the mouth or nose. It allows the doctor to take a direct look at the airways, and can also be fitted with instruments to take samples of mucus or tissue, or to perform minor surgery. The patient is given a sedative and/or local anaesthetic before a bronchoscopy is carried out.

CERVICAL SMEAR TEST

This test detects abnormal changes in cells of the cervix (the neck of the womb). It is performed in order to detect and prevent the later development of cervical cancer. The procedure is simple. It involves wiping off a sample of cells from the cervix which is then sent to a laboratory to check for any abnormal signs. All women are advised to have a smear test at least every three years once they become sexually active.

CHEST X-RAY

A very common test used to show up infection, tumours and other disorders of the lungs. Chest X-rays can also show up heart disorders such as an enlargement of the heart. The X-ray provides an image of the heart and lungs as well as the major blood vessels, bones and joints.

CHOLECYSTOGRAPHY

An X-ray procedure for examining the gallbladder and bile duct to detect gallstones. A contrast medium is given which about twelve hours later finds its way to the gallbladder. X-rays can then be taken. This technique is used much less often now than it once was. Ultrasound scanning can usually confirm a diagnosis of gallstones.

CT SCAN

Computerized tomography scanning, also known as CAT (computerized axial tomography), is a way of producing images of cross-sections (slices) of the body on a screen using very low-dose X-rays and a computer. It is a technique that is especially useful for detecting tumours in the soft tissues of the body and in the brain. CT scanning gives clearer and more detailed information than X-rays used by themselves.

CYSTOSCOPY

An examination of the urethra and bladder using a fibre optic instrument inserted through the urethra. This test is performed to check for tumours of the bladder and for sites of bleeding and infection. Certain bladder disorders can be treated by this method; tumours can be removed and obstructions cleared.

ELECTROCARDIOGRAM (ECG)

A method of recording the electrical impulses that regulate the activity of the heart. It is done by placing electrodes on various parts of the body, which pick up the electrical changes in the heart that take place with each beat. The result is recorded on a paper trace or a screen. Electrocardiography is used to diagnose many disorders of the heart.

ELECTROENCEPHALOGRAM (EEG)

A method of recording the electrical impulses produced by brain activity. It can be used to diagnose certain conditions such as epilepsy, dementia and brain tumour. EEG is also used to monitor the condition of patients who are under general anaesthetic.

Electrodes are placed on the patient's scalp which detect and monitor the different types of brain-waves.

ENDOSCOPY

An examination of a body cavity using a flexible fibre optic instrument with a light-source at one end and a viewing-device at the other (an endoscope). Different types of endoscope are used to examine various parts of the body. A bronchoscope is used to examine the airways, a cystoscope to examine the bladder, a colonoscope to examine the large intestine. Endoscopes may be fitted with a number of different instruments that can take samples of tissue for analysis or perform minor surgical procedures. The patient is usually given a sedative and/or anaesthetic before an endoscopy is performed.

EYE TEST

Eye tests are performed by an optician to check on sharpness of vision and to look for any underlying eye disorders which are often symptomless in the early stages. An optician will examine the appearance of the eyes, lids and surrounding skin and check to see that eye movement is normal. He may check the pressure within the eyeball and also look for abrasions or ulcers on the eye's surface. Tests for sharpness and clarity of vision and colour vision are also part of a full eye test.

HEARING TESTS

Hearing tests are performed to check that hearing is normal, or to determine the amount of hearing loss and, if possible, the source of the problem. Specialized hearing tests are normally undertaken in hospital. There are two main types. Audiometry tests the ability to hear sounds conducted through the air and through the bones of the ear. The test determines the types of sound that the patient has most difficulty hearing. Headphones are used to play sounds of different frequencies which are reduced in loudness until they can no longer be heard.

Acoustic impedance testing can determine the types of damage to the middle earbones and the eardrum which cause deafness. The test uses a special probe containing a transmitter which is inserted into the ear.

INTRAVENOUS PYLEOGRAPHY (Urography)

This is a method of taking X-ray pictures of the urinary system (the kidneys, ureters and bladder). It uses a contrast medium which is injected into the bloodstream and which shows up any obstruction as it works its way through the kidneys and bladder.

The process takes several hours, and X-rays are taken at intervals as the liquid travels through the urinary system.

LAPAROSCOPY

An exploratory operation which allows a doctor to look inside the abdomen for the cause of abdominal illness. The operation is often used to diagnose gynaecological disorders in women. A viewing-instrument called a laparoscope is inserted into a small incision just below the navel in order to view the abdominal cavity.

If signs of disease are found during the exploration, surgery may be undertaken at the same time.

LUMBAR PUNCTURE

A lumbar puncture is a procedure used to take a sample of the fluid that surrounds the brain and spinal cord. It is used to diagnose disorders of the brain such as meningitis, to administer drugs, and to inject contrast medium when a myelogram (see below) is needed. The skin over the lower spine is anaesthetised with local anaesthetic and a hollow needle is inserted between two vertebrae to draw off fluid or to inject drugs.

MAMMOGRAPHY

An X-ray procedure for examining the breast and breast lumps used as part of the screening programme against breast cancer. Mammography allows the detection of small breast lumps before they can be felt and so allows treatment, if necessary, to take place at the earliest stage. The breast is placed between two plates and compressed before being X-rayed. The procedure is painless and takes only minutes.

MYELOGRAPHY

An X-ray examination of the spinal cord and nervous system used to diagnose tumours, disc prolapse, and damaged spinal nerves. A contrast medium is first injected by lumbar puncture, and then X-rays of the spine are taken. CT scans and other more modern imaging techniques are gradually taking the place of myelograms.

RADIONUCLIDE SCANNING

This is a procedure used to discover whether or not a gland or organ is functioning well. It involves a radioactive chemical being injected into the bloodstream. This is absorbed by the organ under investigation, which can then be scanned with a special camera that detects whether or not the radionuclide chemical is being absorbed normally and evenly.

SIGMOIDOSCOPY

An examination of the lower part of the large intestine using an endoscope, a fibre optic viewing-instrument. The endoscope is inserted into the anus to give the doctor a direct view of the rectum and lower bowel. An enema may be given beforehand.

ULTRASOUND SCAN

This is a technique which uses very high-frequency soundwaves to create images of the body's internal organs on a screen. It is commonly used to examine the liver, kidneys and gallbladder, and is especially useful for checking the uterus and the progress of the fetus during pregnancy.

X-RAYS

X-rays produce images of the body's bones, organs or internal tissues through the medium of radiography. Radiography uses carefully controlled electromagnetic radiation to obtain an image on a photographic plate or a fluorescent screen. Bone tissue gives the clearest X-ray picture. Hollow or fluid-filled organs of the body do not show up well unless a radiopaque contrast medium that blocks the X-rays and so shows up tissues is first introduced into the body.

There are a number of specialist contrast medium X-ray techniques used to examine soft body tissues and organs such as the gallbladder, bladder, digestive tract, and the nervous and circulatory systems (see cholecystography, barium X-ray, angiography, bladder function tests, myelography, intravenous pyelography, above).

Even small doses of radiation carry some risk, so X-ray techniques are designed to get the best possible image with the lowest level of radiation.

APPENDICES

APPENDIX 1
Ideal Weight Charts

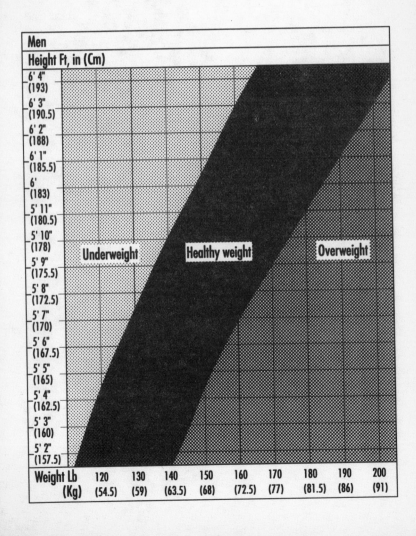

Men									
Height Ft, in (Cm)									
6' 4" (193)									
6' 3" (190.5)									
6' 2" (188)									
6' 1" (185.5)									
6' (183)									
5' 11" (180.5)									
5' 10" (178)		**Underweight**		**Healthy weight**			**Overweight**		
5' 9" (175.5)									
5' 8" (172.5)									
5' 7" (170)									
5' 6" (167.5)									
5' 5" (165)									
5' 4" (162.5)									
5' 3" (160)									
5' 2" (157.5)									
Weight Lb (Kg)	120 (54.5)	130 (59)	140 (63.5)	150 (68)	160 (72.5)	170 (77)	180 (81.5)	190 (86)	200 (91)

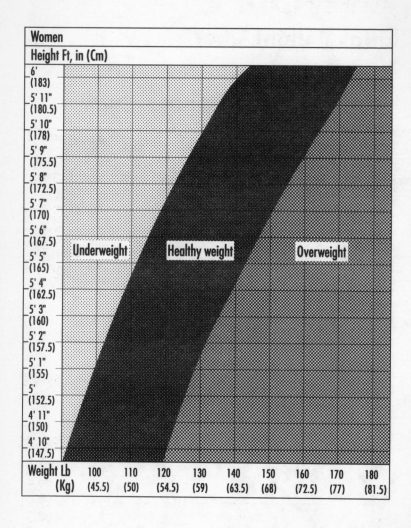

APPENDIX 2
Conversion charts

Average Dimensions of the Premature Baby

Length in cm	Weight in g
26 weeks (14 weeks early) 34 cm	700 g
28 weeks (12 weeks early) 37 cm	900 g
30 weeks (10 weeks early) 40 cm	1250 g
32 weeks (8 weeks early) 43 cm	1700 g
34 weeks (6 weeks early) 46 cm	2000 g
36 weeks (4 weeks early) 47.5 cm	2500 g
38 weeks (2 weeks early) 49 cm	3000 g
40 weeks (on time) 50 cm	3300 g

Measurement Conversion Tables

Centimetres — inches/inches — centimetres
(Inches expressed as decimals, i.e. inches and tenths of inches)

1 cm = 0.3937 inches   1 inch = 2.54 cm

cm	inches	cm	inches	cm	inches
40	15.75	57	22.4	74	29.1
41	16.15	58	22.8	75	29.5
42	16.5	59	23.2	76	29.9
43	16.9	60	23.6	77	30.3
44	17.3	61	24	78	30.7
45	17.7	62	24.4	79	31.1
46	18.1	63	24.8	80	31.5

cm	inches	cm	inches	cm	inches
47	18.5	64	25.2	81	31.8
48	18.9	65	25.5	82	32.2
49	19.25	66	25.9	83	32.6
50	19.65	67	26.3	84	33
51	20	68	26.7	85	33.4
52	20.4	69	27.1	86	33.8
53	20.8	70	27.5	87	34.2
54	21.2	71	27.9	88	34.6
55	21.6	72	28.2	89	35
56	22.0	73	28.7	90	35.4

lb/oz to g – g to lb/oz

1 kg = 2.2 lb   1 lb = 0.45 kg

	5 lb	6 lb	7 lb	8 lb	9 lb	10 lb	11 lb	12 lb	13 lb
0 oz	2270	2720	3175	3630	4080	4535	4990	5445	5895
1 oz	2295	2750	3205	3655	4110	4565	5020	5470	5925
2 oz	2325	2780	3230	3685	4140	4595	5045	5500	5955
3 oz	2355	2805	3260	3715	4165	4620	5075	5530	5980
4 oz	2380	2835	3290	3740	4195	4650	5105	5555	6010
5 oz	2410	2865	3215	3770	4225	4680	5130	5585	6040
6 oz	2440	2890	3245	3800	4250	4705	5160	5515	6065
7 oz	2465	2920	3375	3825	4280	4735	5190	5640	6095
8 oz	2495	2950	3400	3855	4310	4765	5215	5670	6125
9 oz	2525	2975	3430	3885	4340	4790	5245	5700	6150
10 oz	2550	3005	3460	3910	4365	4820	5275	5730	6180
11 oz	2580	3035	3485	3940	4395	4850	5300	5755	6210
12 oz	2610	3060	3515	3970	4425	4875	5330	5790	6240
13 oz	2635	3090	3545	3995	4450	4905	5360	5810	6265
14 oz	2665	3120	3570	4025	4480	4935	5385	5840	6295
15 oz	2695	3145	3600	4055	4510	4960	5415	5870	6320

	14 lb	15 lb	16 lb	17 lb	18 lb	19 lb	20 lb	21 lb	22 lb
0 oz	6350	6805	7255	7710	8165	8620	9070	9525	9980
1 oz	6380	6830	7285	7740	8195	8645	9100	9555	10005
2 oz	6405	6860	7315	7770	8220	8675	9130	9580	10035
3 oz	6435	6890	7340	7795	8256	8705	9155	9610	10065
4 oz	6465	6915	7370	7825	8280	8730	9190	9640	10090
5 oz	6490	6945	7400	7850	8305	8760	9215	9665	10120
6 oz	6520	6975	7430	7880	8335	8790	9240	9695	10150
7 oz	6550	7000	7455	7910	8365	8815	9270	9725	10175
8 oz	6575	7030	7485	7940	8390	8845	9300	9750	10205
9 oz	6605	7060	7510	7965	8420	8875	9330	9780	10235
10 oz	6635	7085	7540	7995	8450	8900	9355	9810	10260
11 oz	6660	7115	7570	8025	8475	8930	9385	9835	10290
12 oz	6690	7145	7595	8050	8505	8960	9410	9865	10320
13 oz	6720	7170	7625	8080	8535	8985	9440	9895	10345
14 oz	6745	7200	7655	8110	8560	9015	9470	9920	10375
15 oz	6775	7230	7680	8135	8590	9045	9495	9950	10405

Temperatures

°F	°C	°F	°C
96	35.6	101	38.3
97	36.1	102	38.9
98	36.7	103	39.4
99	37.2	104	40.0
100	37.8		

Volume of fluids

1 litre	=	1.76 pints
1 pint	=	0.57 litres
1000 cc	=	1 litre
28.4 cc	=	1 oz
20 oz	=	1 pint

APPENDIX 3
Children's development charts

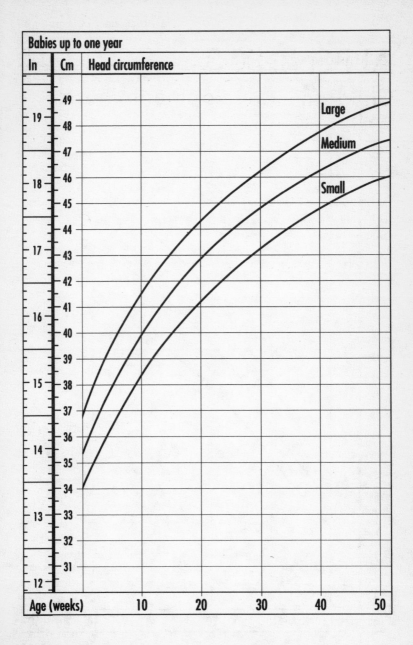

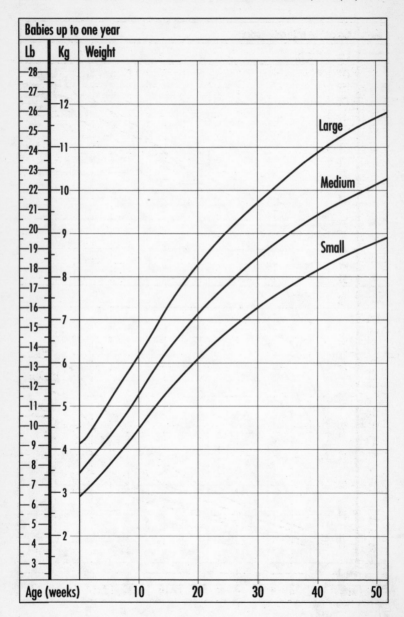

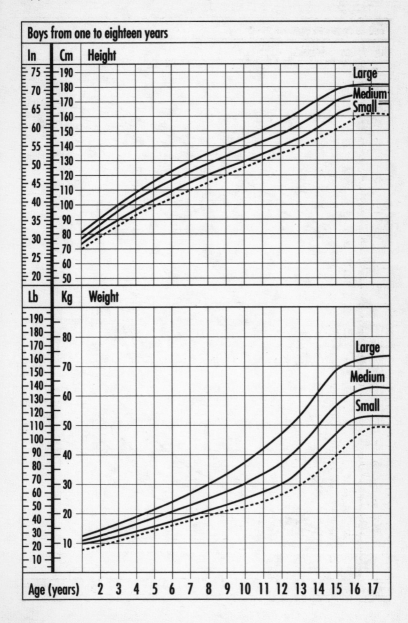

Boys from one to eighteen years

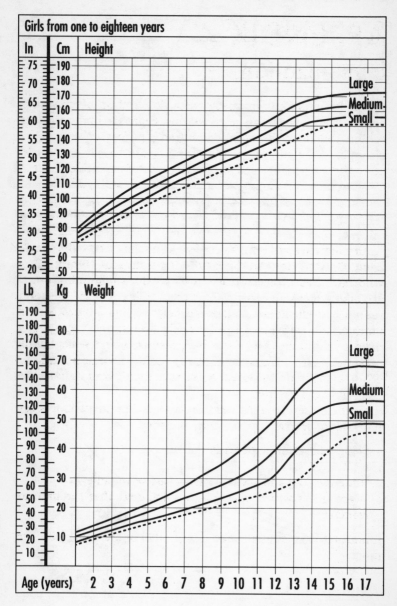

APPENDIX 4
Immunization

Immunization offers your baby protection against infectious diseases, some of which can be dangerous. Thanks to immunization, certain childhood illnesses – diphtheria, polio and tetanus, for example – are now very rare, and diseases such as measles and whooping cough are becoming less common. However, if children are not immunized these diseases will spread again, so it makes sense, for your own child's sake and for the sake of other children, to take advantage of the immunization you are offered.

All children, apart from a very few, can safely receive immunization. Only children who are suffering from acute illness, those who have had a severe reaction to previous immunization, or are taking medicines that reduce their ability to fight infection, should be individually considered before being advised against immunization. Children can be safely immunized even if they have a cold, unless there is a high fever too, and whilst taking most medicines, including antibiotics. Before an immunization is given, a doctor or nurse will make sure that it is all right to give your child the vaccine.

Most children have no reaction at all to immunization. A few have minor reactions which may include:

- being a bit grumpy or grisly
- mild fever
- some swelling and redness on the site of the injection
- slight rashes which may appear some days after the immunization

Immunizations should take place at around the following times.

Two months

First diphtheria, tetanus, whooping cough (all given as one injection), polio (given as drops on the tongue), HIB meningitis.

Three months

Second diphtheria, tetanus, whooping cough, polio, HIB meningitis.

Four months

Third diphtheria, tetanus, whooping cough, polio, HIB meningitis.

Twelve to eighteen months

MMR – measles, mumps, rubella (German measles), given as one injection.

Four to five years

Diphtheria, tetanus, polio, MMR (unless already given), HIB meningitis (unless already given).

Ten to fourteen years

Rubella (girls only), BCG.

Fifteen to eighteen years

Tetanus and polio.

APPENDIX 5
Help yourself to better health

In our increasingly health-conscious society, most of us now accept that a large part of being, and staying, well depends on us. Although our environment and genetic inheritance – our parents! – determine to a certain extent how healthy we are, it's also true that factors such as diet and lifestyle play a most important part in how fit we feel, how well we stand up to the stresses and strains of modern living, and how successful we are in avoiding ill-health.

So what steps can we take to keep ourselves well and healthy? Here are some of the most important ones.

PAY ATTENTION TO DIET

Heart disease, which is the leading cause of death in this country, and certain cancers – of the breast, for example – are linked to a diet high in fats. Cutting down on dairy produce, avoiding too many fried foods, cakes, sausages, pies and fatty meats can dramatically cut your fat intake. There is evidence that eating plenty of fresh fruit and vegetables and other high-fibre foods, such as wholegrain cereals and bread, can give protection against some cancers.

TAKE REGULAR EXERCISE

This will improve the health of your heart and circulation, help to keep the body in good condition, and keep weight down.

AVOID OBESITY

Obesity increases a person's chance of becoming seriously ill. Heart disease, certain cancers, diabetes and other disorders are associated with being obese (more than 20 per cent over maximum ideal weight; see Ideal weight charts, p.xx). If you are seriously overweight, see your doctor and ask for his help in getting back to a normal weight.

GO EASY ON ALCOHOL

Regularly drinking too much alcohol has been linked to some cancers and can cause liver disorders, heart and circulatory problems, and disease of the nervous system. The Health Education Authority recommends an intake of no more than 21 units of alcohol per week for men and 14 for women. One unit equals a small glass of wine, a single measure of spirits, or half a pint of beer.

DO NOT SMOKE

Smoking is the single largest, avoidable cause of ill-health, disease and premature death.

TAKE CARE IN THE SUN

As the damage to the earth's ozone layer increases, so the incidence of skin cancers is rising dramatically. It's sensible to avoid prolonged exposure to the sun and to take careful precautions against sunburn. Wearing a hat and clothing to cover your skin, or applying high-factor suntan creams, lots and often, are important if you are exposed to strong sunlight.

PAY ATTENTION TO CHANGES IN YOUR HEALTH

Be aware of your body.

Any unexplained changes in bowel habit, unusual bleeding, changes in the appearance of a skin mole or wart, unexplained weight loss, persistent cough or hoarseness, should be reported to your doctor.

FOR WOMEN

- Be aware of the normal shape, size and feel of your breasts. Report any unusual changes to your doctor at once
- Take advantage of breast screening. If you are over fifty, a routine mammography under the government National Breast Screening programme is available to you. Keep your appointment when one is offered. Breast screening takes minutes only and saves lives
- Have a regular cervical smear. All women should have a smear at least every three years from the time they become sexually active, and for the rest of their lives

APPENDIX 6
Useful addresses

Age Concern England
  1268 London Road
  London
  SW16 4EJ
  Tel. 081–679 800

National network of community services for the elderly.
  Information service and publications.

Arthritis Care
  6 Grosvenor Crescent
  London
  SW1X 7ER
  Tel. 071–235 0902

Association for Post-natal Illness
  7 Gowan Avenue
  Fulham
  London
  SW6 6RH
  Tel. 071–386 0868

BACUP (British Association of Cancer United Patients)
  121–3 Charterhouse Street
  London
  EC1M 6AA
  Cancer information service, tel. 071–608 1661
  Freephone outside London, tel. 0800 181199
  Counselling service, tel. 071–608 1038

Information, advice and support for cancer patients and their
families.

British Association for Continence Care (BACC)
   Pinewood Studios
   Iver Heath
   Bucks
   SL0 0NH
   Tel. (taped helpline information) 0753 656 716

British Diabetic Association
   10 Queen Anne Street
   London
   W1M 0BD
   Tel. 071–323 1531

British Epilepsy Association
   National Information Centre
   40 Hanover Square
   Leeds
   LS3 1BE
   Tel. (helpline – local rates) 0345 089 599

British Heart Foundation
   102 Gloucester Place
   London
   W1H 4DH
   Tel. 071–935 0185

Useful publications on prevention and treatment of heart disease.

British Migraine Association
   178A High Road
   Byfleet
   Weybridge
   Surrey
   KT14 7ED
   Tel. 0932 352 468.

British Tinnitus Association
  Room 6
  14–18 West Bar Green
  Sheffield
  S1 2DA
  Tel. (helpline) 0345 090210

The Chest, Heart & Stroke Association
  CHSA House
  123–7 Whitecross Street
  London
  EC1Y 8JJ
  Tel. 071–490 7999

CRUSE – Bereavement Care
  CRUSE House
  126 Sheen Road
  Richmond
  Surrey
  Tel. 081–940 4818

Counselling and support for the bereaved.

Disabled Living Foundation
  380–84 Harrow Road
  London
  W9 2HU
  Tel. 071–289 6111

Advice and information on the practical aspects of living with a
disability.

Family Planning Information Service
  27/35 Mortimer Street
  London
  W1N 7RJ
  Tel. 071–636 7866

Information on all aspects of family planning and details of family-planning, menopause, fertility, PMS and other clinics.

Health Education Authority
    Hamilton House
    Mabledon Place
    London
    WC1H 9TX
    Tel. 071—383 3833

Information and booklets on a variety of health topics.

Institute for Psychosexual Medicine
    11 Chandos Street
    London
    W1M 9DE
    Tel. 071—580 0631

MIND: National Association for Mental Health
    22 Harley Street
    London
    W1N 2ED
    Tel. 071—637 0741

Information and advice on all aspects of mental illness and mental handicap.

National Back Pain Association
    31—3 Park Road
    Teddington
    Middx
    TW11 0AB
    Tel. 081—977 5474

Information and support for sufferers of back pain.

National Childbirth Trust
  Alexandra House
  Oldham Terrace
  London
  W3 6NH
  Tel. 071–992 8637

Information, education and support on all aspects of ante-natal care, childbirth and parenting.

The National Eczema Society
  Tavistock House North
  Tavistock Square
  London
  WC1H 9SR
  Tel. 071–388 4097

The National Osteoporosis Society
  Barton Meade House
  P.O. Box 10
  Radstock
  Bath
  BA3 3YB
  Tel. 0761 32472

RELATE (formerly National Marriage Guidance Council)
  Herbert Gray College
  Little Church Street
  Rugby
  Warks
  CV21 3AP
  Tel. 0788 73241/60811

Counselling and support on all aspects of relationships through marriage-guidance clinics around country.

Royal National Institute for the Blind
  Health Department
  224 Great Portland Street
  London
  W1N 6AA
  Tel. 071–388 1266

Royal National Institute for the Deaf
  105 Gower Street
  London
  WC1E 6AH
  Tel. 071–387 8033

Terrence Higgins Trust
  BM AIDS
  London
  WC1N 3XX
  Tel. (helpline) 071–242 1010

Information, support, counselling for people with HIV infection and AIDS and their partners, friends and families.

Women's Health
  52 Featherstone Street
  London
  EC1Y 8RT
  Tel. 071–251 6580

Information and advice on women's health issues.

INDEX OF NAMED ILLNESSES AND CONDITIONS